Preparing for dental practice

Preparing for dental practice

F J Trevor Burke

Professor of Primary Dental Care
University of Birmingham School of Dentistry
Birmingham, UK

Ruth Freeman

Professor of Dental Public Health
Queen's University Belfast
School of Dentistry
Belfast, Northern Ireland

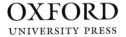

OXFORD
UNIVERSITY PRESS

OXFORD

UNIVERSITY PRESS

Great Clarendon Street, Oxford OX2 6DP

Oxford University Press is a department of the University of Oxford.
It furthers the University's objective of excellence in research, scholarship,
and education by publishing worldwide in

Oxford New York
Auckland Bangkok Buenos Aires Cape Town Chennai
Dar es Salaam Delhi Hong Kong Istanbul Karachi Kolkata
Kuala Lumpur Madrid Melbourne Mexico City Mumbai Nairobi
Sao Paulo Shanghai Taipei Tokyo Toronto

Oxford is a registered trade mark of Oxford University Press
in the UK and in certain other countries

Published in the United States
by Oxford University Press Inc., New York

A catalogue record for this title is available from the British Library

ISBN   0198508646 (Pbk)

10 9 8 7 6 5 4 3 2 1

Typeset by Cepha Imaging Pvt. Ltd., Bangalore, India
Printed in China
on acid-free paper by Phoenix Offset Ltd.

Preface

Preparing for dental practice is for senior dental undergraduate students and vocational dental practitioners to prepare them for dental practice. It is also for general dental practitioners to enable them to undertake continuing professional development. The value of this book is its holistic flavour, combining the business of practice with the science of clinical dentistry and the humanity of patient care. Readers will be able to prepare for dental practice in the 21st century by amalgamating these aspects of primary care in order to care for their patients.

The majority of undergraduate texts in the UK specialise in oral surgery, preventive dentistry, endodontology, crowns and bridges, and routine conservative treatment. Increasingly, UK (and US) dental schools are providing comprehensive patient care programmes and general practice courses. In these courses, students are encouraged look at the holistic care of the patient and identify their overall treatment needs, rather than thinking purely in a clinical and departmental manner. In order to develop an holistic view of dental care, the first chapter of this book examines issues in relation to career choices, the location of the practice, and the means by which access to dental care may be increased. Chapters 2 and 3 take the reader inside the dental practice to examine relationships within the practice setting. This includes the relationship with the patient as well as the dental team. The fourth chapter describes clinical excellence in primary dental care by examining clinical decision-making, the need for referral, and the place of prevention and restorative philosophies in the treatment of patients. The last chapters examine the business of dental practice and suggest future pathways for the newly qualified dental practitioner.

Preparing for dental practice is new and exciting and provides the background for an holistic approach to patient care and treatment. It does this by encouraging senior dental undergraduates, vocational dental practitioners, and general dental practitioners to inquire and investigate their role as primary dental care practitioners. It provides accessible information to enable dentists to enjoy their primary dental practice, and to experience a successful career in primary dental care.

Acknowledgements

Dr Mike Grace

Dr Robin Gray

Mr Colin Lee

Professor G R Ogden

Professor A J M Plasschaert

Professor A Richardson

Mrs Penelope Vasey

Professor N H F Wilson

Many thanks are also due to Mrs Lyn Malthouse for her expert secretarial assistance.

Contents

Contributors

Dr Mike Grace
Editor
British Dental Journal
64 Wimpole Street
London
W1M 8AL, UK

Dr Robin Gray
62 Manchester Road
Altrincham
Cheshire
WA14 4PJ, UK

Professor Graham Ogden
Dundee Dental School
Park Place
Dundee
DD1 4HN, UK

Professor Alphonse Plasschaert
Department of Cariology and
Endodontology
Katholieke Universiteit Nijmegen
PO Box 9101
NL 6500 HB Nijmegen
The Netherlands

Professor A Richardson
33 Cherryvalley Park
Belfast B7 56PN
Northern Ireland

Mrs Penelope Vasey
53 St Helens Wood Road
Hastings
East Sussex
TN34 2QR, UK

Professor Nairn Wilson
Central Office
GKT Dental Institute
Floor 18, Guy's Tower
King's College London
Guy's Hospital
London
SE1 9RT, UK

1 The first job

1.0 CAREER OPTIONS

While it could be considered that a career in dentistry is limited by the fact that the new graduate is trained only as a dentist, there is indeed a wide variety of careers within dentistry itself (Table 1.1).

A suggested pathway for these career options is illustrated in fig. 1.1. This is derived from the Faculty of General Dental Practitioners' (UK) career pathway, which provides a route to Fellowship of the Faculty and provides for recognition of general dental practitioner special interests. In this respect, the Faculty of General Dental Practitioners (UK) provides postgraduate education and training for general dental practitioners (GDPs), and produces guidance on issues such as record keeping and prescribing (www.fgdp.com).

Table 1.1 Career options within dentistry

General dental practice	Salaried practice
Principal (practice owner)	in industry
Associate	in the armed forces
Assistant	with a corporate body
Vocational dental practitioner	Community dental clinic
Specialist	Personal dental service (PDS)
	Academia
	Hospital dentistry

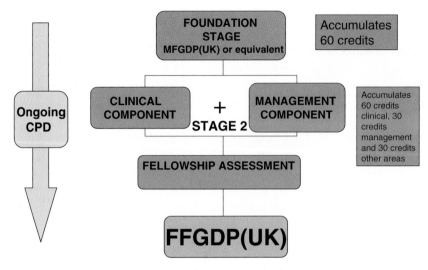

Figure 1.1 FGDP(UK) Career Pathway.

1.1 GENERAL DENTAL PRACTICE (PRIMARY DENTAL CARE)

The vast majority of dentists in the UK work in a dental practice or primary dental care environment. There is the opportunity to purchase a practice, which permits the dentist to be his/her 'own boss' as much as is possible within any career. The practice principal chooses the materials to be used, the décor of the waiting room, the equipment in the surgery, and, even, the patients that s/he doesn't want to treat! Alternatively, a dentist may elect to be an associate or assistant, with less involvement in the administration of the practice.

Associateships and assistantships

The purchase of a practice generally demands that the purchaser intends to be fixed in the practice location for a period of time, in order to build a rapport with the patients and develop the practice. Consequently, until a dentist is certain about the location in which they wish to practice, or until they are in a position to raise the funds with which to purchase a practice, a dentist may wish to become an associate or assistant.

The term *associate* is peculiar mainly to the UK. In broad terms, the associate in a practice contracts to pay the practice owner (practice principal) a proportion of his/her gross fees, usually in the range of 50–60% (depending on location and demand, among other factors), once laboratory expenses have been subtracted. In return, the practice principal agrees to supply staff, materials and equipment, and usually patients, and to maintain the practice premises and equipment. The practice principal will often expect the associate to make an agreement that the goodwill of the patients remains with the practice principal. While it is not unusual for associates to remain in the same practice for many years, there is no long-term financial commitment to remain in the same location. An associateship has therefore been the method of employment, for many, before purchasing a practice and making a long-term commitment to a particular practising location.

An *assistant* is often employed on a salaried basis, treating the practice principal's patients. Within the NHS (National Health Service), an assistant will generally work, by prior arrangement, within the contract between the principal and the NHS.

Vocational training (Mrs Penelope Vasey)

Applying for a VDP position

Vocational training, as organised in the UK, is unique in the world of dentistry. In this scheme, new graduates undertake Vocational Training (VT) in selected training practices, where they work four days per week, with one day per week being allotted to postgraduate education. The majority of Vocational Dental Practitioners (VDPs) go straight into vocational training upon graduation. A number of them will have first worked in hospital, but opportunities and salary are equal for everyone undertaking vocational training in practice.

The Dental Vocational Training Authority website will direct you to the geographic location of your choice: English Deaneries, Wales, Scotland and Northern Ireland. Trainers are appointed by competitive interview, together with a rigorous inspection of their practices. VDPs can be confident that training practices are of a high standard, and that Trainers have been appointed for their suitability to support and guide you through your introduction to practice: the VT year. It is possible to undertake vocational training part time, if you have domestic or serious sporting commitments. The vast majority of schemes start in August each year, and the trainer lists are published via the Dental Vocational Training Authority towards the end of March or beginning of April. A smaller number of places are available to start in January or February.

There are generally sufficient places for every new UK graduate, and feedback from past VDPs advises the new graduate to choose carefully and limit his/her application to a few practices that appeal to the applicant. Having identified a number of suitable practices, the applicant for a VDP position may ask for the opportunity to visit the practice. It should be made clear whether the visit is informal, or for a formal interview. Ideally, the applicant should try to visit during working hours, to get a feel for the atmosphere and meet the support staff. Some deaneries run 'job shops' when the new graduate can meet a number of Trainers face to face, in one location.

Past VDPs say that the best aspects of the VT experience are:
- the relationship with the Trainer, in the training practice
- support at Study Day sessions with peers and Adviser

Thus it is of prime importance to choose a practice that is suitable, rather than jumping at the first available opportunity. There is no greater chance of securing a position by applying to a large number of practices, and this will only serve to put you under extra pressure at a stressful time. DVTA runs a clearing system in July when more places become available through failures at the final BDS examination.

Having been offered a position and having decided to accept it, the VDP and the potential Trainer will be required to sign a 'letter of intent'. This is to safeguard both parties. The Trainer agrees not to offer the job to anyone else, and the applicant agrees to stand by his/her acceptance. A contract of employment cannot be signed whilst still a student, but once the dentist has graduated and is on the Dentists Register, the VT contract may be signed. This document sets out the terms and conditions of employment as a VDP, including hours of work: 35 per week in the practice, or 28 hours when time is spent away at a study day. Details of four weeks' holiday entitlement, sick and maternity leave are all covered. The VDP is also required to sign an Educational Agreement with the Postgraduate Dean or Director. This clearly lays out the VDP's responsibilities in attendance and in keeping the Professional Development Portfolio.

Full time vocational training lasts for 365 days, and attendance at all the 30 study days is compulsory in order to gain a certificate of completion of vocational training.

What will the VDP learn during the VT year that will prepare him/her for practice?

The curriculum includes a range of topics which will prepare the VDP well for practice as an assistant or associate, and provide him/her with an appreciation of all the knowledge and skills required as a practice owner. Confidence building in clinical skills is important in the early part of the VT period. Invaluable advice and support will be given by the Trainer in treatment planning and managing patients. The VDP will learn how to work in a team and supervise support staff, and liaise with laboratories, hospitals and general medical practitioners. Some topics may seem to have little relevance at this time, but an introduction to health and safety issues, staff management, financial issues and employment law will prove critical to the future practice owner. Finally, experience in the training practice and discussion at study days will provide an informed idea of what to look for in a practice. Having spent a year in an approved training practice, the VDP will probably be less willing to accept any compromise in practice standards in the future. For example, Trainers are required to provide the VDP with a trained dental nurse. Having experienced the benefits of good chairside assistance, this will probably be a high priority when looking at future jobs.

Whilst most study days will be at the scheme's postgraduate centre, there are opportunities for visits to national events and organisations. A trip to London may take in the General Dental Council, British Dental Association or one of the Defence organisations. The experience of attending a national conference or study day of the Faculty of General Dental Practitioners is a valuable part of the VT experience. These occasions will vary from year to year, chosen by the VT Advisers for relevance to VDPs.

On a daily basis the Trainer offers close support to the trainee. Besides being available in the practice a minimum of three days per week for help on demand, s/he is required to spend time each week on a tutorial. Although the Trainer and trainee will plan the topics to be covered, this is the opportunity to discuss clinical problems that have occurred in the surgery. Schemes consist normally of 12 training pairs, and are run by a Vocational Training Adviser. The Adviser is a source of experienced help, as well as organising the study day sessions and facilitating problem solving sessions within the group of VDPs. Feedback shows this to be considered the single most beneficial aspect of VT.

Within each Deanery a Regional Adviser coordinates the schemes, organises training for trainers and is generally responsible for the operation of VT locally. Finally, the Postgraduate Dean or Director carries the ultimate responsibility for the training that is delivered, supports the other VT personnel and signs the certificate of completion of VT. S/He has the power to require VDPs to undertake a further period of training if attendance at either the practice or study day sessions has been inadequate.

How will I know if I am making progress?

An integral part of VT is the Professional Development Portfolio (PDP). This document belongs to the VDP. Before starting clinical work the VDP will agree with the Trainer and record a tailor-made programme in the PDP. This is a unique opportunity to gain extra experience in clinical areas in which the trainee may lack confidence, or even where the VDP knows that they are weak. By recording week by week the things that have gone well, or not so well, and by building up clinical experience, VDPs can look back and see tangible evidence of progress. Here is a way also of ensuring that the Trainer gives as much time and support as is needed. Of course as the year wears on, needs will change, as will the speed of clinical work and management of patients.

At the end of the VT year, the certificate of completion of vocational training is the passport to automatic granting of a VT number when applying to join a Health Authority list. The successful VDP may then become a principal in the General Dental Services, working on his/her own list number. However, VDPs have been heard to say that to view VT as a means merely to obtaining a VT number is to miss out on a unique opportunity to learn alongside an experienced Trainer and be truly prepared for practice. As with most things in life, the more you put in, the more you will get out.

The financial change from VDP to associate

For the VDP who becomes an associate, a word of warning. The VDP is a salaried position. As an associate, the dentist must wait for patients to pay their accounts or for the third-party insurers (for example, the National Health Service) to pay the fees that are claimed. This may often take two to three months. During that time, the associate will receive no, or very little, fee payments. This is a situation which must be planned for, for example, by appraising the bank of the situation and negotiating an overdraft. The converse is that fee payments will continue after leaving the associate position.

'High street' specialists

Although the majority of general dental practitioners (GDPs) provide all of the treatment which their patients require, there is also, within the practice environment, an opportunity to specialise, or to have an interest in one particular form of treatment. This could lead to referrals from outwith the practice, or from other dentists within the practice. The route to becoming recognised as a specialist requires the dentist to take the MFDS qualification from one of the Royal Colleges, followed by three years' training in a Specialist Registrar post in a hospital environment. A more complete description of specialist training has been provided by Ibbetson (2003).

1.2 SALARIED PRACTICE

Dentists may opt to enter salaried practice in a variety of locations. The advantages of such practice could be the predictable salary in comparison to that in general dental practice which is subject to fluctuations depending on busyness, holidays, etc. Salaried practice may also have fixed hours of work.

Locations for salaried practice include industry, where large companies provide a dental service for employees (Industrial Dental Service) and the Armed Forces, with the potential for travel to the different world locations where forces are deployed. Corporate bodies may also employ dentists on a salaried basis, although some also employ dentists under associate arrangements.

1.3 COMMUNITY DENTAL SERVICE

The Community Dental Service (CDS), which employs dentists on a salaried basis, provides a varied service to several specific groups of the community. Once thought of as the 'School Dental Service', it provides screening and care (if required) to child patients, the elderly and patients with special needs. The CDS provides a safety net service (Freeman *et al.* 1997) for those unable to access care in the usual way. There is a clear career structure, from dental officer (specialist) to director of community dental services (management). It has a well-developed programme of postgraduate training, with a high proportion of its dental staff achieving a postgraduate qualification.

1.4 PERSONAL DENTAL SERVICE (PDS)

Prior to 1997, National Health Service (NHS) dental services in the UK could only be delivered by general dental practitioners on the basis of a national contract and a nationally negotiated scale of fees. Personal Dental Services (PDS) were initiated following recommendations in a number of reports, including the report by Sir Kenneth Bloomfield in January 1993 in which the exploration of alternative methods of remunerating general dental practitioners was suggested, partly as a response to growing problems with the availability of NHS dental care.

After consultation with the dental profession, it was announced that the local commissioning of general dental services would be explored through pilot schemes, with dentists' entry into these schemes being voluntary. PDS is an alternative method of delivering NHS dental services, based on local contracting arrangements, with the contract for dental services being agreed between the local health authority and one or more providers of dental services. PDS Pilots use the flexibility of locally negotiated contracts to tackle local problems related to dental services and oral health, and it may be considered that local contracting may produce more sensitive and responsive dental care.

A central feature of the PDS initiative is the piloting of new ways of funding primary dental care. PDS pilots, in general, have developed two main remuneration models, a salaried model and a capitation system. Another feature of PDS pilots was expected to be their use of Professionals Complementary to Dentistry (PsCD). Some PDS pilots may become a model for new local contracting arrangements if proposals whereby Primary Care Trusts become responsible for arranging contracts with the dentists working on the NHS in their area, are instituted.

1.5 ACADEMIC DENTISTRY

An academic career in dentistry is usually associated with a university post in a teaching school. The majority of dental academics will maintain a clinical

Table 1.2 Principal activities of a dental academic

Teaching	Administration
• Undergraduate	• Organisation of courses
• Postgraduate	• Student care
Research	• Committees
• Clinical	**Writing**
• Laboratory	• Research papers
Clinical	• Review articles
• Patient treatment	• Books
• Chairside teaching	• Peer reviewing
Examining	
• Undergraduate	
• Postgraduate	
• Research Theses	

interest and work with patients both in their own clinical practice and also by way of chairside teaching. However, a smaller number of dental academics choose to work purely in research or in the pre-clinical part of the dental undergraduate course.

The principal activities of a dental academic are shown in Table 1.2.

Teaching

Teaching may form a substantial part of a dental academic's job (Scott 2003). This will take the form of lectures and seminars or problem-based learning, but will generally include the chairside supervision of students providing patient treatment. Most dental academics will also provide teaching at postgraduate level, either in the form of lecture courses or 'taught' higher degree (e.g. Masters) courses.

Research

Research is an important aspect of the dental academic's work. The dental academic will normally be expected to have achieved an MSc degree by research in the earlier part of their career, followed by a PhD, which would generally be considered essential for promotion to higher academic positions. The type of research undertaken will depend upon the expertise and equipment available in the institution in which the academic is employed, but it is essential that the topic(s) for research are actually of interest to the individual, because it may be considered that the researcher will approach his/her work with a good deal more enthusiasm if the subject stimulates the individual. Research may be carried out in a wide number of areas (Scott 2003). These include clinical research (such as clinical trials of materials, preventive programmes or assessment of disease levels) or laboratory-based research (such as dental materials testing, molecular and cellular biology).

Clinical

Dental academics, other than those involved in the teaching of pre-clinical dental students, will normally hold an honorary hospital appointment and will undertake treatment of patients, often those who are referred from GDPs. Most dental academics develop their own special clinical interest and may carry out clinical research based around their treatment of patients, having obtained ethical approval if necessary.

Examining

Examinations are central to the dental undergraduate course and postgraduate diplomas, so the dental academic will be involved in these as an examiner but, often, also as the co-ordinator of the examination. S/He will also be called upon to examine research theses.

Administration

Administration comes with most walks of life, and the dental academic is not exempt from this in relation to courses to be arranged and committee work, notwithstanding the preparation of the often voluminous documentation by which courses and research are assessed.

Writing

It is essential that research findings are disseminated to the end users – dentists and patients, and, accordingly, the writing of research abstracts (for presentation at research meetings) and papers is central to the role of the dental academic. S/He may also choose to write review articles or books, usually on a subject on which s/he has particular expertise, as this is also a valuable method for dissemination of information.

The peer review process, by which articles in peer-reviewed journals are assessed and checked for accuracy prior to publication, is central to the publication of good 'evidence', and as dental academics are often experts in their own fields of interest, they tend to carry the main burden of the peer review process. Some may also become the editor of a dental journal.

1.6 HOSPITAL DENTISTRY

The ultimate aim of a dentist entering the hospital service will generally be to achieve the position of Consultant. Currently, the MFDS diploma awarded by the Royal Colleges in the UK is the entry qualification required for specialist training as a consultant in a dental speciality, of which 13 are recognised by the General Dental Council (GDC) (Table 1.3).

Completion of specialist training allows the trainee the choice of achieving a hospital consultant position or entering specialist dental practice in the 'high street'. Both positions lead the specialist to treat a comparatively narrow range of albeit more complex conditions when compared with his/her GDP colleagues and the majority of cases treated by the specialist will be referred from GDPs or medical practitioners. The hospital specialist will be responsible for the teaching of the trainees and for administering the service in his/her department. The hospital consultant and specialist trainees should also undertake research, and due to their extensive patient throughput, this may take the form of assessments of treatment provided. Those dentists who are trained to specialist level may make the choice between hospital or 'high street' by virtue of the salary conditions, namely salaried in the hospital and fee per item in practice.

2.0 APPLYING FOR A POSITION

Prior to applying for a position, it is essential that the prospective candidate writes a curriculum vitae.

2.1 WRITING A CURRICULUM VITAE (CV)

Why write a CV?
- A CV is often all that is requested when applying for a post
- It shows a degree of organisational and computer skill
- It gives the applicant an opportunity to tell others how good s/he is

---

Table 1.3 Specialities for which the GDC maintains a specialist register

Oral Medicine	Oral Surgery
Orthodontics	Dental and Maxillofacial Radiology
Restorative Dentistry	Prosthodontics
Pediatric Dentistry	Endodontics
Dental Public Health	Periodontology
Oral Microbiology	Surgical Dentistry
Oral Pathology	

A CV should provide evidence of suitability for the post advertised as well as giving an overview of the applicant's life and interests.

CV layouts may vary according to the post being applied for – for a research position, for example, the applicant may highlight that aspect of his/her career. For the purpose of this book, however, it will be assumed that the applicant is applying for his/her first position. Attractive presentation and absence of typographical errors are important. Ideally for a first position, the CV should be no more than 3 pages of A4 in length.

Essential information to be included on a CV are:

Personal details

This section should include given name, surname, date of birth, marital status (number of children) and address. For the dental student, there may be value in stating both home and term-time addresses, with all telephone numbers, and e-mail address if the applicant picks up his/her e-mails regularly.

Education and academic achievements

This should include secondary schools and university education, listing grades at A-level and examinations passed as an undergraduate.

Prizes and distinctions

This should list major prizes and distinctions at school and university or as part of general interest (such as Duke of Edinburgh's Award).

Positions of responsibility

These are often unpaid positions, which indicate the writer's enthusiasm and lack of apathy. Examples of positions which could be included are treasurer of student society, captain in sport, and, editorship of student review.

Interests, hobbies, and activities

This section may provide the considerate interviewer with a starting question and should be interests in which the candidate plays an active part. Genuine achievements should be included, such as grades at music, membership of drama groups and/or choirs.

Personal statement

The applicant should give a personal statement giving details of their aspirations and ideals, for example, stating how much s/he is looking forward to working hard, to working in general dental practice, to achieving high quality, etc.

Other details

This section could include details of research elective projects completed, previous positions (for the person who has undertaken other work prior to becoming a dental student) or special clinical interests or clinical modules undertaken. Again, this may often provide an easy starting question for the interviewer.

References

Persons chosen to provide references should have recent knowledge of the applicant and be relevant for the position applied for. In this respect, therefore, for hospital posts, the referee should, ideally, be in a hospital position, while for a dental practice post, the referee could be a part-time lecturer/GDP and a senior member of the academic staff who has supervised the applicant in the clinic. The applicant should always ascertain whether a potential referee is happy to provide a reference before their name is included on the CV. A referee should decline the opportunity to provide a reference if:
- they do not know the applicant sufficiently well, or,
- if they are unable to write something constructive about the applicant.

It is worth asking a potential referee for the best way of making urgent contact, for example at home or by mobile phone, as the competition for some positions may be intense and a quick phone conversation to the referee may provide the person who has advertised the position with the information that s/he needs, rather than waiting for the delivery of letters etc., thereby facilitating the early appointment of the applicant.

2.2 THE LETTER OF APPLICATION

The covering letter, with the CV, will give the person who placed the advertisement a first impression of each applicant. While in the past it could be considered that a neatly handwritten letter was appropriate, a neat, computer-generated letter (and neatly written envelope) is now the norm. The letter should be addressed to the practice owner by name or hospital/university personnel manager. Your name should be printed under your signature.

This letter should include the following:
- The reason why you have applied for the advertised post
- The features in the advertisement which attracted you to that particular post
- How the post fits your overall career plan
- When you are available for interview

2.3   THE FIRST INTERVIEW

Dental students entering professional practice will normally have to undertake an interview with their potential employer. This may often take the form of an informal 'tour' of the practice and/or a more formal interview. The interview will normally be conducted by the practice owner, but, on occasions may be delegated to the practice manager, if one is employed. There are two sides to an interview:

- first, the interviewer will wish to determine the suitability of the interviewee for the advertised position, and,
- second, the interviewee will want to obtain the maximum amount of information about the practice and its modus operandi.

Either way, it is incumbent on the interviewee to present his/herself to the best advantage, and to 'sell' (but not oversell) him/herself. The interviewee should be honest, but should strive to tailor his/her answers to give the best impression. However, the interviewee is always potentially in a difficult position, as it is the interviewer who is in control of the proceedings.

The interviewer will wish to ascertain the suitability of the candidate for the position, and, for a VDP position, to determine whether the candidate and the practice owner and his/her team will be able to happily work together for a period of a year (or more if all goes well and the VDP is offered an opportunity to continue as an associate). The practice owner will also seek to determine the candidate's communication skills and his/her ability to work with others. The interviewer may also seek to determine the candidate's clinical knowledge by asking for answers to a variety of clinical questions. Answers should be 'to the point' and prior experience at dental school recounted in a positive manner. However, the candidate's success or failure will be largely due to how well they talk and present themselves at interview. Nevertheless, the interviewee should consider him/herself as an equal, although the candidate will be less experienced.

For the interviewee, advance preparation is important. The interviewee should ask the practice owner to send the practice's patient information leaflet, which should contain information which is relevant to the interview. There is merit in taking a look at the outside of the practice prior to the interview, to gain information about the practice location, if the candidate does not already know the area. Additionally, this will mean that the interviewee is less likely to get lost when attending for the interview and s/he will know how long the journey to the practice will take. A look at the Dentists Register will reveal the year and place of graduation of the practice owner/interviewer and will thereby give the interviewee an estimate of the interviewer's age.

The candidate should write a list of the questions to which s/he wants answers, and bring this to the interview. These could include:

- Will the candidate be taking over a full list of patients from the previous dentist, and, if not, how many new patients attend the practice per week?

(There would appear to be little point in taking a position in a practice which has insufficient patients: there can be few experiences less rewarding than sitting in a dental practice with nothing to do but read the newspaper!)

- Can I have a look at the present dentists' appointment books?
- What are the practice opening hours?
- What are the arrangements for treatment of emergencies outside normal working hours, and how often will the candidate, if successful, be on call for these?
- What proportion of patients return regularly for recall, what is, in general, the attitude and oral health of the practice's patients?
- Is there freedom to choose materials and laboratory?
- Who is responsible for bad debts?
- What is the general practice policy for acceptance of NHS patients?
- Is the practice owner a member of organisations such as the British Dental Association or the Faculty of General Dental Practitioners?
- How much CPD does the practice owner undertake and what are his/her special interests?
- Is the candidate's surgery fully equipped, with light curing unit, emergency oxygen and emergency kit?

For candidates attending for associate or assistant positions, the candidate should additionally enquire about the financial arrangements pertaining to the position. For a VDP position, the candidate should additionally enquire about the number of patients that s/he will be expected to treat each day, what subjects will be covered in the tutorials, and whether the practice has had a trainee previously.

Additionally, and importantly, the interviewee should seek to speak with the dentist who is leaving the practice, in an effort to determine his/her reasons for leaving and to ascertain how (un)happy s/he has been while working at the practice. There would also appear to be value in finding out details of staff turnover by speaking to members of the staff: a high rate of staff turnover could be considered to indicate a less-than-ideal working environment.

Interviews, from the viewpoint of the interviewer, are discussed in Chapter 3 Section 1.5. page 102.

2.4 THE FIRST IMPRESSION

The candidate should be neatly dressed, clean cut and conservatively dressed. Ideally, both men and women should wear a suit. Taking care over appearance not only shows respect, but also will demonstrate to the interviewer that the candidate considers the interview and the position important. If perfume or aftershave is worn, this should not be applied in excess. Fingernails should be clean. On meeting the practice owner, the candidate should give a firm hand-shake, make (and then maintain) eye contact and smile.

Further reading

The British Dental Association has produced a wide range of Advice Sheets (Table 1.4) and Patient Leaflets. Those entitled, 'Getting a job', and 'Which way now?' and 'A guide to careers in dentistry' are especially valuable to final year dental students applying for their first position.

3.0 CHOOSING THE 'RIGHT' PRACTICE

Dentists may often spend as many hours in their dental practice as they may spend with their family or on recreation (fig. 1.2). Time spent on choosing the

---

Table 1.4 The British Dental Association produce a wide variety of Advice Sheets which are free to members. Examples, which may be relevant to dental students or recent graduates, are:

Buying and selling a practice
Health and safety law for dental practice
Marketing in dentistry
Associate agreements
Employing an assistant in dental practice
Corporate dental practice
Radiation in dentistry
Infection control in dentistry
Computers in dental practice
Setting up in practice
Ethics in dentistry
Data protection
Prescribing in dental practice
Collecting money from patients
Introduction to taxation
Fee setting in private dental practice
Staff recruitment
Working abroad
Vocational training in dental practice
A guide to General Dental Services Regulations
Religious and cultural diversity – helping to improve awareness in dentistry
CPD, clinical audit and peer review
Help with overseas electives

> **46 working weeks per year**
> **5 working days per week**
> **8 working hours per day**
> **= 1840 working hours per year**
> **= 32% of *WAKING* hours!**

Figure 1.2

practice best suited to an individual's aspirations, talents and interests is therefore time well spent. It is always tempting to accept the first job offer, but there are strong indications for the new graduate or prospective associate to evaluate the character and philosophy of the practice in which a position is vacant. Questions asked at interview or at an informal 'look' around the practice (see below) may be invaluable in preventing misunderstandings later. For a vocational dental practitioner, associate or assistant, it should be ascertained that the patient base is assured. However, above all, both parties should try to ascertain whether they will be able to co-habit within the same premises for whatever the period of time.

There is considerable merit, therefore, during the final undergraduate year, to have visited a number of practices, so that experience is built up in assessing the pros and cons of the practices visited prior to a first job or prior to vocational training.

The character of any given practice is a function of a variety of factors, some of which are interdependent. Among these are:

• Location
• Social class of patients
• The practice philosophy
• The practice staff
• The practice décor
• The practice equipment
• Whether a dentist lives on the practice premises
• Number of dentists
• Emphasis on postgraduate achievements and continuing professional development
• The practice organisation

3.1 PRACTICE LOCATION

City centre location

The patient base of a city centre dental practice is likely to be different from that of a practice in the town or city suburbs or in rural locations. The city centre practice will generally attract patients who work in the city, and is therefore unlikely to have a significant proportion of children and adolescents. Many specialist practices are located in the city centre, as they are likely to attract patients from a wider catchment area than the typical general dental practice and will therefore require a central location. There will often be a high concentration of practices in a small area. Referral to a specialist practice, dental school or hospital from a city centre practice is likely to be simpler from a logistical point of view than from a practice in a more remote situation. It is also likely that the city centre practice will be accessible to the dental laboratory, with the advantages that the dentist can readily discuss mounted study casts etc., or refer patients to the laboratory for shade taking should the need arise.

Other advantages of the city centre practice may be the close proximity to theatres and places of entertainment, but disadvantages may include problems with parking or its high expense. Furthermore, as rental or purchase costs will be higher in the city centre than in the suburbs, the practice will often not be at ground floor level and will therefore not be likely to attract 'passing' patients.

For the practitioner who enjoys treating paediatric patients and whole families, therefore, the city centre practice is unlikely to be suitable.

Suburban location

The suburban practice is more likely to attract families of patients, with the typical scenario being mother and children attending for routine check-up appointments in a 'block' booking. A dentist who not only enjoys treating children but enjoys carrying out a wide range of treatments for adults and children should therefore investigate practices in a suburban location. Referral for specialist care is also likely to be straightforward from a suburban practice. If the practice is located on a main road or on a bus route, potential patients passing by the practice may be attracted to it – 'passing' patients who could be a source of new patients if the practice is on the ground floor, or otherwise readily visible by those passing.

The comments above regarding liaison with the dental laboratory also apply to the suburban practice.

Rural location

The practice in a rural location is likely to attract patients of all ages and walks of life, given that they are likely to choose the practice based on accessibility rather than other factors. The treatments in such a practice are likely to be more varied than in other types of practice, especially if referral for specialist care is difficult logistically. It may therefore be desirable that the practitioner in a rural practice undertakes additional training in, for example, removal of impacted third molars, or orthodontics. The latter is possibly of the greatest relevance, given the need for frequent visits, often spread over a period of a year or more. The dentist in a rural practice is likely to become a well-known local figure in the community in which s/he works. This may hold advantages, but, on the other hand, may mean that their every action is scrutinised!

Disadvantages may include remoteness from the laboratory, reluctance of patients to accept referral to a remote surgery or hospital and difficulties for the staff in travelling to centres of postgraduate education.

Working in socially deprived or affluent areas

The 1998 UK Adult Dental Health Survey, as with its predecessors, has illustrated differences in attitudes to dental treatment and attendance between different social groups. Patients from a background where the head of the household is of social class IV or V are less likely to attend a dentist regularly, may be less appreciative of the benefits of maintaining dental health and may be inclined to attend only when in pain than those from households where the head is in social groups I, II or III (higher socio-economic status groups), (Kelly *et al.* 2000). The practice in an area where the predominant social groups are IV or V (lower socio-economic status groups) may therefore have a higher incidence of patients failing to attend for appointments. Conversely, the satisfaction which the operator may gain when s/he has successfully improved the oral health of a previous non-attender may be great. Higher socio-economic status (SES) group patients may attend on a more regular basis, but may also have higher expectations from treatment, which may be unjustified. Higher SES patients have a greater oral health awareness, but there is no guarantee that their oral health behaviours (toothbrushing) will be better than those from lower SES groups.

3.2 THE PRACTICE PHILOSOPHY

Patient expectations of dental treatment have increased over recent decades, and it may be considered that the majority of patients, today, would prefer to retain, rather than lose teeth. It is difficult to understand how a dentist with an extraction, rather than restorative and preventive philosophy, can be successful in practice at the present time. However, while this is an extreme example, the practice philosophy could embrace a reluctance to try new techniques, purchase new equipment or become fully computerised. Good clinical practice demands that dentists and other healthcare professionals stay abreast of current thinking and to question the 'evidence' that is presented in the literature and advertising. The ideal practice philosophy should be forward-looking and therefore encourage learning, audit and research.

Patients are increasingly discerning and it should be remembered that dentists are, to some extent, in competition with each other. Patients will therefore eventually discover the practice philosophy. The practice providing contemporary restorative and preventive treatments of high quality at a reasonable cost will ultimately become more successful than the practice which does not.

The age of the practice owner is not necessarily a factor which influences the practice philosophy, given that the older practitioner can add experience to the 'evidence' for success.

For the student or dentist assessing the philosophy of the practice that they are considering joining, a few well-chosen questions may help, for example:

Q: Do you fit many resin-retained bridges here?

A: No. We tried those some years ago but they don't work, do they?
(Indicative of questionable practice philosophy)

Q: Do you fit many resin-retained bridges here?

A: We fit them when there is a strong clinical indication, but our practice audit has shown that the occlusion is a big factor in the success of these restorations. We give a five-year unconditional guarantee when there is an edge-to-edge occlusion or minimal overbite. We like to provide minimally invasive treatments where possible.
(Indicative of good practice philosophy)

3.3 THE PRACTICE STAFF

Nurses and receptionists

The dentist not only provides treatment but also brings management skills to the practice: s/he will be judged by the painless-ness of injections, by the appearance of restorations and dentures, by the lack of pain or problems post-treatment and by 'chairside manner'. However, it is arguably the remainder of the dental team who give the practice much of its image. (See The Dental Team Chapter 3, Section 1.0, p 94.) All staff should be neatly and tidily dressed, ideally in uniforms. The reception staff should have an air of quiet efficiency. Too much unnecessary conversation shows that they are not as busy as they should be, or answering the telephone as rapidly as they should. All staff should be helpful: their attention should be centred on the patient. Telephones should be answered quickly. In the surgery, the nursing staff should be considerate to patients, the majority of whom are probably not where they want to be when they visit a dental surgery! They should also be efficient and quiet (it is easy to make loud noises which may startle patients when transferring instruments from one site to another!) and know where the various instruments, devices and materials are kept.

Number of dentists

A practice with more than one dentist will, by the nature of the situation, have more than one set of ideas about any given topic. In most circumstances, that will be beneficial. The greater number of dentists in the practice, the less frequent will be the on-call emergency times and the less likely that an inexperienced dentist will be left in the practice alone to cope with problems – clinical and administrative – that arise.

When visiting a practice the staff morale may be judged by asking the number of years that staff members have been employed at the practice. A high turnover of staff is generally an indication of poor staff morale, poor pay or conditions and a less-than-ideal working environment. It is worth noting that unhappy staff perform less well and more grudgingly than happy, contented and valued staff.

Questions for the potential VDP or associate to ask staff in a practice

Q; How long have you worked here?
A: Three months, and I'll be glad to get away
   (Indicative of low staff morale)
Q; How long have you worked here?
A: I've been here for three years and I'm the shortest serving staff member.
   (Indicative of good staff morale)

Another indicator of the practice staff and image:
Phone the practice as though you were a new patient: Was the phone answered promptly and courteously? Would you like to be attending that practice yourself, if you were a patient rather than a dentist?

3.4   THE PRACTICE DÉCOR

Decorative tastes and styles are personal and it is therefore impossible to please everyone. However, the dental practice is a workplace and as such the décor should be functional. The waiting room should be decorated in a relaxing style, and adequate numbers of up-to-date magazines should be available, as too should tea or coffee. Informative dental literature should also be available, possibly with explanatory videos etc. It should be comfortable, but not overly so because patients will not normally expect to be kept waiting in the waiting area for excessive periods of time. Any patient kept waiting in the waiting area should expect an explanation from the reception staff. An overcrowded waiting area is indicative of either a practice whose number of surgeries has grown without a corresponding increase in the size of the waiting area, or of dentists who are not running to schedule. Neither are to be commended.

Above all, all areas of the practice should be clean and tidy. Patients will feel that a dirty practice is likely to also be less than fastidious about matters of instrument sterility. Untidiness indicates a lack of organisation, again, not something which enhances patient faith in the procedures of the practice.

3.5   THE PRACTICE EQUIPMENT

New surgery equipment is such a high capital expense that it is something which the average dentist, in a practising career of 40 years, will only purchase three or four times. It is therefore unreasonable to expect that surgery equipment should be new. Moreover, it is likely that when a practice owner purchases new equipment it may be for his/her own surgery, with the older equipment being transferred to the assistant's or associate's surgery. However, it is reasonable to expect that the equipment will be in good decorative and working order, that sufficient handpieces are available (likely to be four or five, depending on patient throughput) and that all other surgery equipment, such as the light curing unit, is in the surgery rather than being shared with another surgery in the practice.

A not unreasonable question to ask is:

Q: I particularly like brand MM bonding agent. Will the practice purchase it for me?

A: No we only use XX because it's cheapest.
   (indicative of a penny pinching attitude)

A: Yes. We will be delighted to learn about the new bonding agents that you were taught about at dental school.
   (indicative of a positive attitude)

3.6   WHETHER A DENTIST LIVES ON THE PRACTICE PREMISES

The practice owner living on the premises is not an unusual situation in the UK. It presents advantages and disadvantages to the practice owner. For the owner, advantages include no travel to work and ease of access to home and family during the working day. Disadvantages include the lack of 'winding-down' time between workplace and home and the fact that patients may perceive the dentist as being always available. Depending on how separate the practice is from the house, the new associate VDP or assistant may have particular problems in changing the practice environment. With the wrong personalities, it may seem like entering a family rather than a practice.

3.7 EMPHASIS ON POSTGRADUATE ACHIEVEMENTS AND CONTINUING PROFESSIONAL DEVELOPMENT

While the failure to achieve postgraduate qualification is not necessarily indicative of a poor practice, or a working environment in which professional development will be difficult, the achievement of one or more postgraduate qualifications by the dentists in a practice is a certain endorsement of the desirability of continuing postgraduate development. Such a practice is likely to encourage their members of staff to take time off for postgraduate courses. Attendance at meetings and courses is an essential aspect of a professional person's life and development, notwithstanding the fact that patients will expect their dentists to be abreast of latest developments. Furthermore, the person who has achieved a dental degree at one time generally requires the mental stimulation that postgraduate study may bring. The practice which actively encourages such study, and which provides a good library of peer-reviewed journals is to be sought after.

The achievement of additional qualifications should not be confined to the dentally qualified members of the team. It is just as important for the nursing staff, practice manager and hygienists to enrol for continuing education as part of their continuing development.

3.8 THE PRACTICE ORGANISATION

The smooth everyday running of a practice is central to the enjoyment of work by all in the practice. Enjoyment of work by the staff will make for a happy practice and this, in turn, will be noticed by patients.

There are many facets to practice organisation and the reader should consult a text on practice management for a full appraisal of the subject. However, organisation is dependent on all staff in the practice being aware of their responsibilities and of the policy of the practice team on matters relating to everyday matters or emergencies. Some of these responsibilities and policies are best placed in written form. Examples of practice policy which could be in written form include matters as varied as:
- policy on infection control,
- on needlestick injuries,
- on late cancellations,
- on postgraduate education by all members of the team,
- on non- or late-payment of fees,
- on the patient who attends late for an appointment,
- on whether certain items of treatment are available within the NHS regulations or whether certain patient groups will be treated within the NHS,
- whose responsibility it is to check the currency of the emergency drugs, or,

- the responsibilities of the various members of the team in the event of a patient collapse.

Committing such policies and responsibilities to paper makes it simple for joining members of staff to be made aware of the hows and wherefores of the practice organisation. In all matters of practice organisation it is essential that written protocols are available, for three essential functions:

- first, writing a protocol forces the writer to gather his/her thoughts together
- second, the written protocol can be discussed with other members of the dental team and the agreed protocol amended in the light of new information/techniques
- third, the and may be used for training existing and new members of staff

Staff – or team – meetings are a valuable forum for interaction between all in the practice and it is at these meetings (see The Dental Team, Chapter 3, Section 1.7, p108) where policies may be discussed and formulated, or changed. Such team meetings should be sacrosanct in the appointment book, and may best be held outwith the practice building so that discussions may be made without the potential for interruption.

3.9   THE PATIENT BASE

It is essential that the new graduate or potential associate seeking a position knows whether there is a patient base already registered with the practice which is sufficient to keep them employed, and in the case of an associate, with the potential to achieve the income which is desired. While the new dentist in a practice will ultimately hope to attract new patients to the practice, s/he needs a list of patients to treat on week one. The person hoping to work in a practice should therefore be given full access to appointment books, to check on practice busyness. Enquiries should be made on the number of new patients attending the practice per month, and a well-organised practice should be able to provide such figures. It should also be noted that an associate will generally treat more patients than a vocational dental practitioner, so a VDP's list will not be as large as that for an associate.

At the outset, the new dentist in a practice should be aware whether s/he is taking over a 'list' from a previous dentist or whether s/he will be expected to build up a new list of patients. The latter situation is likely to arise when a dentist starts up a new practice, but should not what a VDP or associate would expect.

While the arrangements for a VDP are relatively fixed, for the potential associate there are a number of questions to be asked. Among these are:

- Financial arrangements – % of gross paid to the practice owner
- Assignment of fees – to practice owner or associate
- Who pays bad debts?
- Holiday entitlement

Questions to be asked by both VDP and associate are:
- Is there a choice of laboratories or is the practice tied to one laboratory?
- Is there freedom to order materials that are preferred?

4.0 EASE OF ACCESS TO DENTAL TREATMENT

Among the factors upon which access to dental treatment depends are:
- Physical access
- Psychological access
- Financial access

4.1 PHYSICAL ACCESS

The issues of physical access to dental treatment involve:
- the ability of the patient to travel to the practice: this in turn, is dependent on whether the practice is conveniently located to the patient's home or place of work, whether the patient has his/her own transport, or, if not, whether they can justify the cost of a taxi or other public transport
- the accessibility of the practice itself: whether ramps are provided for wheelchair users or the infirm, whether a lift is available if the surgery is not on the ground floor, and whether car parking is easily available.

In this regard, an information sheet should be available, not only for fit and able patients, but also for those with special needs. Written directions to the practice from a variety of directions, or a map, should be included.

4.2 PSYCHOLOGICAL ACCESSIBILITY

In 'Maintaining Standards: Guidance to Dentists on Professional and Personal Conduct' (GDC 1997) the General Dental Council stated that:

> 'Dentists have a duty to provide and patients have a right to expect adequate and appropriate pain and anxiety control' and that included

> 'Pharmacological methods of pain and anxiety control, local anaesthesia and conscious sedation techniques'

The need to provide oral health care which affords anxious patients the opportunity to access dental treatment in the usual way is recognised as a goal of primary dental care. The requirement for dental practitioners to increase psychological accessibility is associated with the formation and maintenance of the treatment alliance (see Chapter 2, Section 1.3: the dentist–patient relationship). In order for dentists to achieve this accessibility and treatment goal there are a number of behavioural management and pharmacological techniques which may be employed. It must be emphasised that the role of behavioural management and pharmacological methods of anxiety control should be directly related to the quality and quantity of the dental anxiety experienced by the patient. The means of assessing dental anxiety and the choice of behavioural management and/or pharmacological technique used is described in greater detail in Chapter 2.

Behavioural management techniques to increase psychological accessibility:

- **Iatrosedation** is, simply, dentists providing the environment to allow for effective communication between the patient and themselves. Iatrosedation is the first part of the psychological management of the dentally anxious patient. A non-clinical setting allows the dentist to establish rapport and for the patient to express their fears and worries.
- **Tell-show-do** is a simple means of preparing children and anxious adults for dental care. Tell-show-do reduces anticipatory anxiety by providing patients with details of their treatment. The dentist tells the patient what is to be done, shows the patient what will be done and then does it. Communication is an important aspect of this behavioural technique with the dentist using language the patient can understand. In terms of evidence-based treatment tell-show-do have been shown to reduce anticipatory anxiety in children attending for DGA extractions (Carson and Freeman 1998).
- **Desensitising hierarchy** is a process in which the patient and dentist jointly negotiate a treatment plan based on the patient's least feared item of dental treatment through to their most feared. Treatment starts with the least feared treatment (e.g. prophylaxis) and works through those items of treatment which are slightly feared (e.g. infiltration anaesthetic and filling) to the most feared (e.g. an extraction of a lower molar). During the treatment the patient's confidence increases as their anxiety is reduced. As before communication is central to this form of behavioural management as it allows the dentist and patient to work together towards a common treatment goal. In essence the patient's dental anxiety is contained and reduced prior to progress to the next treatment in the hierarchy.
- **Hypnosis, biofeedback and relaxation** are a family of behavioural techniques which are used to reduce anxiety by inducing muscle relaxation:
  - i. **Hypnosis** induces an altered state of consciousness which is characterised by muscle relaxation and suggestion. Hypnosis has been used extensively in dentistry to reduce anxiety and induce states of relaxation. Disadvantages however exist as patients who are extremely anxious find it harder to relax and enter the hypnotic state and the technique is time intensive with new patients.

The British Society for Medical and Dental Hypnosis (BSMDH) is a national organisation of doctors, dentists and other health professionals within the NHS. The BSMDH offers recognised and accredited training for those health professionals interested in hypnosis and its use in the treatment of stress/anxiety. For those interested in this therapeutic technique, more information may be sought from the BSMDH website (http://www.bsmdh.org).

ii.   **Relaxation** or applied relaxation (Willumsen *et al.* 2001) is associated with biofeedback and hypnosis. The principle behind relaxation is that physical relaxation inhibits anxiety. The dentally anxious patient will be instructed to tense and then relax muscles throughout the entire body which will lead to relaxation of the body as a whole. Relaxation has been shown to be an excellent means of helping patients reduce their dental anxiety. It is also a useful adjunct to the treatment of patients with severe gagging reflex.

iii.   **Biofeedback** involves the training of patients to control their physiological responses (e.g. increased heart rate) to anxiety-provoking situations. The technique is based on the premise that through monitoring the patient can voluntarily control the physiological manifestations of anxiety and by doing so can reduce the emotional dimension of anxiety.

Pharmacological techniques to increase psychological accessibility

• **Oral sedation:** Benzodiazepines are the most commonly used group of drugs for pre-medication. The disadvantages of oral sedation with diazepam include the difficulty in monitoring serum levels, the onset of action for oral diazepam is 45–90 minutes with a duration of action of 2–4 hours. Other benzodiazepines include midazolam. The advantages of midazolam are that it has a shorter half-life, rapid onset and duration of action. Beta-blockers have been used with little success in reducing dental anxiety.

• **Inhalation sedation** or relative analgesia (RA) is the combination of nitrous oxide with oxygen. The 'hypnotic effect' of RA is enhanced by the dentist's communication skills. RA is recognised as being the most controllable and safest technique of conscious sedation currently available to the dental profession. The main advantages of RA are well known: these include the ease of administration, titratability, reversibility, rapid induction and rapid recovery. RA has been shown to be effective and successful in reducing anxieties, acceptable to child patients and cost-effective. General dental practitioners regard RA as an acceptable means of treating anxious children but have called for continuing education to increase their clinical competency in the administration of inhalation sedation (Freeman and Carson 2003).

• **Intravenous sedation:** Many agents are used for intravenous sedation but the most common are midazolam and propofol. The intravenous sedation can only occur when a separate sedationist is present who can devote his/her attention and time to the level of consciousness of the patient.

4.3 FINANCIAL ACCESS

The ability of a patient to pay for their treatment is a fundamental aspect of access to treatment. To some, the cost of treatment may be a barrier to care. Dentists are in the top 5% of wage earners in the community, and it therefore follows that dental treatment may seem expensive to the remaining 95%. In the UK, treatment is funded in a variety of ways.

NHS treatment

A considerable proportion of the population of the UK opt to receive their dental treatment within the NHS regulations. At the time of writing patients pay up to 90% of their treatment costs up to a maximum amount. Patients may be exempt from these charges if their salary falls below a certain level. Expectant mothers and those who have had a baby within the previous year are also exempt. Arguably it is the group whose salary falls just above the exemption level who will find funding for NHS – or, indeed, any form of dental treatment most difficult.

Private treatment

This may take one of two forms:
(i) the patient pays the fee for each item of treatment
(ii) the patient enters a private capitation scheme such as Denplan (Denplan Ltd. Winchester, UK) to whom they pay a fixed amount per month. The scheme, in turn, provides the majority of their treatment at no additional cost. The amount which the patient pays is set following an assessment of their potential treatment needs, which is assessed from their previous incidence of treatment.

A considerable proportion of the population of the UK, variously assessed at between 25% and 50%, do not attend for regular dental examinations. Some patients choose to attend only for emergency treatments. Others do not attend because of anxiety about dental treatment. Others do not attend because they feel that treatment is not affordable. Others prefer to spend their disposable income on other things, perceiving dental treatment (or oral health) to be of limited value.

In the UK, in 2002, *circa* 25% of treatment was carried out privately by the ways described above (Laing and Buisson 2003), with the UK public being estimated to have paid, for the first time, more funds for private treatment

(£1.9 billion) than for NHS treatment (£1.8 billion). It may be considered that this figure is increasing annually.

NHS fees are negotiated on a national basis between representatives of the dental profession and government, and, accordingly, in areas of the UK in which dental practice premises, staff wages and running expenses are high, many dentists have ceased to provide dental treatment under the NHS. In these areas, those who are low wage earners may find difficulty in obtaining dental treatment which they feel is affordable. A number of initiatives have been commenced by the government to improve access to NHS dentistry. Among these are the Personal Dental Services pilots (see Section 1.4).

Financial access: The dentist's viewpoint (see section on dentist–patient relationship)

From the dentist's viewpoint, fees per item of treatment are generally calculated on the basis of the time required to complete the treatment at a given hourly rate, that rate being decided by the dentist. Within the NHS, the hourly rate is fixed following negotiations between the profession and government. For private treatment, the hourly rate comprises (see also section on finance):
- The dentist's time charge for the treatment, plus
- The overheads in running the practice on a daily basis.

> The highest proportion of the overhead costs is generally the staff wage cost, followed by charges associated with the premises (bank loan for purchase of premises and equipment, or, capital cost or rental, local charges, electricity, materials, stationery etc.), dentist and staff pensions.

The situation may therefore arise in which the dentist feels that the fees awarded by the NHS do not cover his/her hourly rate. In such a situation, for the practice to remain viable financially, there are only two courses of action:
- Cease treatments under the NHS
- Carry out the treatment in a shorter time.

In the latter situation, it does not always follow that treatment carried out faster is less good than treatment carried out slowly. Some dentists are capable of working faster than others. However, it is generally when a dentist feels that s/he is not carrying out the treatment to his/her best ability because of insufficient time that can be awarded because the dentist's hourly rate is greater than that awarded by the NHS, or because laboratory fees are limited, or that s/he is not able to offer the most appropriate treatment, that the dentist opts to no longer treat patients under the NHS conditions. It will be apparent to readers that this situation is most likely to be reached by dentists practising in the most expensive areas of the UK where practice running costs are likely to be highest. Hence, a proportion of practices in the UK, perhaps a quarter (Laing and Buisson 2003) have 'converted' wholly to private treatment or partly NHS and partly private. This 'conversion' may be a difficult decision for the dentist, who may be giving up the financial security of working for the NHS, to enter the different demands that providing private treatment brings and the uncertainty of how many patients will 'convert' from NHS to private. However, the dentist should never judge a patient's ability to pay for treatment. Patients from lower SES groups may value their dental care sufficiently to pay private fees for it; conversely, higher SES group patients may have the attitude that they deserve NHS treatment because they pay substantial monies in taxes. Additionally they may be unable to afford private care because they have children at private school, a high mortgage and the 'need to keep up with the Jones'. Alternatively, they simply may not value their oral health.

5.0 EMERGENCIES IN THE DENTAL SURGERY: EQUIPMENT AND DRUGS

Prevention of emergencies

Medical emergencies are best prevented. All members of the dental team should be trained to be watchful for signs of patient collapse (for example, sweating and skin pallor) in all areas of the practice, including non-clinical areas. Additionally, emergencies may be prevented by careful assessment of the patient prior to and during treatment. All members of the team should know how to clear and maintain the airway and be competent in carrying out cardiopulmonary resuscitation (CPR). Records of initial training and update courses (annual or more frequent refresher courses are appropriate) should be kept. Additionally, dentists should be able to perform venepuncture.

Medically compromised patients should be identified by ascertaining their medical history. New patients should complete a comprehensive written medical history and this should be verified verbally, with the medical history updated at each subsequent course of treatment.

All dental practices should have clear protocols for the treatment of medical emergencies which may arise, for use in staff training.

Common causes of collapse in the dental surgery

Fainting

Fainting may be caused by anxiety/fear, pain, fatigue, fasting and high temperature and humidity. The patient will feel weak or nauseated, skin pallor will be evident and the skin will be cold and moist. The pulse will be slow initially, then fast and full, and the patient may lose consciousness.

Treatment is by lowering the head and loosening tight clothing. Recovery is normally rapid; if not, other causes of collapse should be considered. A glucose drink or tablet may be given if the patient has not eaten, and oxygen administered to medically compromised patients.

Angina

Angina is caused by a reduction in oxygen to the heart through narrowing of the coronary arteries, or high blood pressure which leads to increased oxygen demand and may increase the size of the heart. The patient will experience a severe 'crushing' pain which may radiate down the left arm: it will be brought on by exertion, anxiety or during digestion of a large meal and will be relieved by rest. Treatment is by stopping activity or treatment, administering glyceryl trinitrite tablets or spray sublingually, and providing oxygen. If the symptoms do not subside in 10–15 minutes, the patient diagnosis should be revised to coronary thrombosis.

Coronary thrombosis/myocardial infarct

A myocardial infarct occurs when a branch of the coronary artery is blocked by a clot causing death of the muscles supplied by that artery. The patient will experience pain in the chest, radiating down the left arm, with the pain of much longer duration than angina. There will be signs of shock, such as cold clammy skin and low blood pressure. These symptoms may occur in a patient with no previous cardiac history. Management is first by calling for help from the emergency services (with a view to obtaining admission to hospital), placing the patient in a comfortable position, administering oxygen at 2–4 litres per minute. In cases of cardiac arrest, CPR should be commenced.

Epilepsy

This is a convulsive disorder, with the attack being characterised by an aura, a tonic phase in which the patient loses consciousness, may stop breathing and become rigid. This is followed by a clonic phase in which convulsions occur. The patient may traumatise their tongue in either phase. Management is by stopping treatment, attempting to prevent the patient from harming him/herself, and placing the patient in the recovery position after the clonic phase. Fits generally stop spontaneously. After the fit, the patient may feel drowsy and should be accompanied home. Prevention is by ensuring that patients take their medication as usual prior to treatment.

Collapse of patient taking steroids

Steroids are prescribed for a wide range of medical conditions and adrenal function may be depressed in patients taking steroids for one month or more. Symptoms include weakness, nausea and pallor, weak and rapid pulse and loss of consciousness. Management is by placing the patient flat, administering oxygen, summoning assistance and giving 100 mg Hydro-cortisone sodium succinate IV and obtaining urgent transport to hospital. Prevention is typically by pre-operatively doubling the dosage of medication for patients taking less than 7.5 mg prednisolone per day who require surgery or extended treatment. It is advisable to liaise with the prescribing physician.

Anaphylaxis

This is a severe allergic reaction characterised by a sudden and catastrophic release of histamine. In the dental surgery, most common causes are penicillin or latex allergy. Symptoms include facial oedema, bronchospasm and difficulty in breathing/wheezing, severe shock, nausea and vomiting and progressive loss of consciousness. Management is by laying the patient flat, summoning urgent assistance, giving 0.5–1 ml 1:1000 adrenaline IM (smaller doses for younger patients), repeating this dose every 15 minutes, Hydrocortisone 100-200 mg IM slowly, 10–20 mg chlorpheniramine maleate (Piriton) 10 mg/1 ml slowly IV, administering oxygen and obtaining urgent transport to hospital.

Asthma

An acute asthmatic attack may be triggered by the stress of a visit to a dental surgery, infection or allergens. Symptoms include breathlessness, expiratory wheezing and a rapid pulse. Treatment is by reassurance and the administra-tion of the anti-asthma drugs normally taken by the patient, such as a salbu-tamol nebulizer, which the patient should be asked to bring when attending the dental surgery. If the attack is severe, assistance should be requested and 200 mg hydrocortisone IV administered.

Hypoglycaemia

The insulin-dependent diabetic may develop hypoglycaemia by missing a meal while taking their normal dose of insulin. Emotional stress may also compound the problem. Symptoms include drowsiness, excitability and aggression, sweating and trembling and a full and rapid pulse. Management is by laying the patient flat, giving sugar orally if the patient is conscious and 1 mg Glucagon in 1 ml sterile water IM if the patient is unconscious. The unconscious patient should be transferred to hospital.

Hyperventilation

Hyperventilation may occur in cases of anxious or hysterical overbreathing. Symptoms include lightheadedness, agitation and paraesthesia. Manage-ment is by reassurance, and breathing into a bag. If the hyperventilation is severe and the patient does not respond to the measures outlined above, then it may be necessary to give 10 mg diazepam IV.

Cerebral vascular accident (Stroke)
This may occur with a cerebral thrombosis, haemorrhage or embolus. Symptoms include loss of consciousness, headache, deep and noisy breathing, incontinence and paralysis of one side of the body. Management in the dental surgery is by maintenance of the airway, administration of oxygen and transfer to hospital at the earliest opportunity.

Inhaled or swallowed object
Foreign bodies, such as teeth, crowns or root canal instruments, may be swallowed or inhaled. A patient may exhale the foreign body without stimulating the cough reflex. If it is suspected that a foreign body has been swallowed or inhaled, the patient should be transferred to hospital for a chest or abdominal X-ray. Further management depends upon whether the object is in the lungs or gut, and whether it is sharp or blunt. The Heimlich Manoeuvre may be performed if the patient is choking and unable to cough out the foreign body.

From the above, it can be seen that a typical dental practice emergency drug cabinet may contain a wide variety of drugs (Table 1.6). A system

Table 1.6 Typical emergency drugs which may be stored in a dental practice

Drug	Presentation	Route of administration	Indication
Oxygen	Cylinder, valve, tubing and mask	Inhalation	All emergencies except hyperventilation
Glyceryl trinitrate	0.4 mg per dose spray	Sublingual	Angina
Adrenaline	1 mg in 1 ml (1:1000)	IM	Anaphylaxis
Hydrocortisone sodium succinate	100 mg in 2 ml sterile water	IM	Anaphylaxis advenal crisis Asthma
Chlorpheniramine maleate	10 mg in 1 ml solution	IM	Anaphylaxis
Glucagon	1 mg powder + 1 ml sterile water	IM (epipen)	Diabetic hypoglycaemia (patient unconscious)
Glucose	Drinks or tablets	Oral	Diabetic hypoglycaemia
Salbutamol inhaler	0.1 mg per dose	Inhalation	Asthma

(after Thornley A: course work submitted for MSc at University of Birmingham and British Dental Association Practice Quality System) should be in place which gives a staff member responsibility for checking that the drugs which are stored are within their use-by-date.

6.0 INFECTION CONTROL

The application of a risk-free infection control regimen is central to the safe treatment of patients in dental practice. All dentists have a duty of care to their patients to ensure that adequate infection control procedures are followed. Members of the dental team have a duty to ensure that infection control procedures are followed routinely. The mouth carries a large number of potentially infective micro-organisms; saliva and blood are known vectors of infection. Most carriers of latent infection are unaware of their condition and it is important, therefore, that the same infection control routine is adopted for all patients.

The British Dental Association produces a wide variety of Advice Sheets for dental practitioners, including one on practice infection control. The most recent version of this was published in 2003 and is reproduced in Sections 6.1 to 6.33 of this chapter, by kind permission of the British Dental Association.

6.1 INTRODUCTION

Infection control in health care continues to be the subject of intensive research and debate. This advice sheet condenses current knowledge and recommendations in a practical form for the dental practitioner.

Implementing safe and realistic infection control procedures requires the full compliance of the whole dental team. These procedures should be regularly monitored during clinical sessions and discussed at practice meetings. The individual practitioner must ensure that all members of the dental team understand and practise these procedures routinely.

Every practice must have a written infection control policy, which is tailored to the routines of the individual practice and regularly updated. The policy should be kept readily available so that staff can refer to it when necessary.

6.2 ROUTINE PROCEDURES

A thorough medical history should be obtained from all patients at the first visit and updated regularly. Medical history questionnaires alongside direct questioning and discussion between the dentist and the patient are recommended. Discussions should be conducted in an environment that permits the disclosure of sensitive personal information. The medical history information should be retained as part of the patient's dental records.

The medical history and examination may not identify asymptomatic carriers of infectious disease and universal precautions must be adopted. This means that the same infection control procedures must be used for all patients.

6.3 PATIENT PERCEPTION

As a result of frequent media coverage, the public is now aware of the need for dentists to practise good infection control. Displaying an infection control statement may be appropriate in your practice to help allay patient anxiety and gain them confidence. It may encourage them to ask questions, so never be too busy to give an answer. Ensure that all the members of your practice staff are confident and competent to answer patients' queries or know whom to refer to when necessary.

6.4 ACCEPTANCE OF PATIENTS

Whilst a health professional has the right to accept or refuse to treat a patient, it is important that the dental profession accepts the responsibility of providing dental treatment to all members of the community. Dental clinicians have a general obligation to provide care to those in need and this should extend to infected patients who should be offered the same high standard of care available to any other patient.

Those with Human Immuno-deficiency Viruses (HIV), who are otherwise well, and carriers of the hepatitis viruses may be treated routinely in a primary care setting (general dental practice, community dental service, for example). The evidence indicates that, in the absence of an inoculation injury, the risk of infection to a dental health care worker during the dental treatment of HIV-infected individuals is negligible. HIV-infected individuals need a high standard of dental care when they are asymptomatic to minimise dental problems. If they subsequently develop Acquired Immune Deficiency Syndrome (AIDS) it may be appropriate for them to be referred for specialist advice and care.

It is unethical to refuse dental care to those patients with a potentially infectious disease on the grounds that it could expose the dental clinician to personal risk. It is also illogical as many undiagnosed carriers of infectious diseases pass undetected through practices and clinics every day. If patients are refused treatment because they are known carriers of an infectious disease, they may not report their conditions honestly or abandon seeking treatment; both results are unacceptable. Those who reveal that they are infected are providing privileged information.

6.5 CONFIDENTIALITY

All information disclosed by a patient in the course of medical history taking, consultation and treatment is confidential. No part of the information obtained should ever be disclosed to any third party, including relatives, without the patient's permission. Dentists are responsible for the security of information given by patients, whether it is written on record cards or held on computer. All members of the dental team should be aware of the duty of strict confidentiality and seek to ensure it at all times. It is strongly recommended that practices have a confidentiality policy in place and that contracts of employment for dental staff include a statement on the need to maintain confidentiality.

6.6 THE INFECTED DENTAL HEALTH CARE WORKER

All health care workers have an overriding ethical and legal duty to protect the health and safety of their patients, and those who carry out exposure-prone procedures should be immune to or non-infectious for hepatitis B (page 11). A dental clinician who believes he or she may be infected with a blood-borne virus or other infection has an ethical responsibility to obtain medical advice, including any necessary testing. If a clinician is found to be infected, further medical advice and counselling must be sought. Changes to clinical practice may be required and may include ceasing or restricting practice, the exclusion of exposure-prone procedures or other modifications. An infected clinician must not rely on his/her own assessment of the possible risks to their patients. Failure to obtain appropriate advice or act upon the advice given could lead to a charge of serious professional misconduct.

Exposure-prone procedures are those invasive procedures where there is a risk that injury to the worker may result in exposure of the patient's open tissues to the blood of the worker. These include procedures where the worker's gloved hands may be in contact with sharp instruments, needle tips and sharp tissues (spicules of bone or teeth) inside a patient's open body cavity, wound or confined anatomical space where the hands or fingertips may not be completely visible at all times.

A dentist who employs a dental nurse who is subsequently found to be infected with a blood-borne virus must undertake a risk assessment to determine whether there is a risk to patients and whether the dental nurse should be redeployed within the practice. The risk assessment must take into account the duties performed by the dental nurse and the likelihood that the infection could be transmitted to a patient or another member of staff. An infected dental nurse must not undertake exposure-prone procedures in order to remove, as far as is possible, the risk of transmitting infection.

There may be employment issues that need to be considered and advice should be sought from the employment advisers at the BDA.

The following recommendations for infection control procedures in routine dental practice are made in light of current knowledge and may be subject to revision, as further information becomes available.

6.7   TRAINING IN INFECTION CONTROL

All dental staff must be aware of the procedures required to prevent the transmission of infection and should understand why these procedures are necessary. Regular monitoring of the procedures is essential and the infection control policy for the practice should be reviewed regularly and updated when necessary.

All new staff must be appropriately trained in infection control procedures prior to working in the practice. Training should equip staff to understand

- how infections are transmitted
- the practice policy on decontamination and infection control
- what personal protection is required and when to use it
- what to do in the event of accidents or personal injury.

6.8   SURGERY DESIGN

The layout of the surgery, which should be simple and uncluttered, is an important aspect of infection control. There should be two distinct areas: one for the operator and one for the dental nurse, each with a washbasin, which should have elbow- or foot-operated taps, and liquid soap dispensers. The operator's area would have access to the turbines, three-in-one syringe, slow handpiece, bracket table and operating light. The dental nurse's area would contain the suction lines, perhaps the three-in-one syringe, curing light, all the cabinetry containing dental materials and a designated area for clinical waste disposal and the decontamination of instruments.

Clean and dirty areas within the surgery should be clearly defined. Where possible, instruments should be decontaminated away from the surgery in a room containing the autoclave(s), ultrasonic bath(s), instrument washer(s) and sinks and a separate hand wash basin. If instruments are cleaned manually before sterilisation, the sink must be of sufficient depth to enable instruments to be fully covered with water during cleaning to minimise the risk of splashing.

6.9 VENTILATION

- The surgery should be well ventilated; usually an open window will suffice but, in some cases, it might be appropriate to install an extraction fan or air conditioning
- ventilation systems should exhaust to the outside of the building without risk to the public or re-circulation into any public building
- the recommended fresh air supply rate of ventilation systems should not fall below 5–8 litres per second per occupant and should not create uncomfortable draughts
- mechanical ventilation systems must be regularly cleaned, tested and maintained according to the manufacturer's recommendations to ensure they are free from anything that may contaminate the air
- recycling air conditioning systems are not recommended.

6.10 FLOOR COVERING

- The floor covering should be impervious and non-slip. Carpeting must be avoided
- the floor covering should be seam-free; where seams are present, they should be sealed
- the junctions between the floor and wall and the floor and cabinetry should cove or be sealed to prevent inaccessible areas where cleaning might be difficult.

6.11 WORK SURFACES

- Work surfaces should be impervious and easy to clean and disinfect – check with manufacturers on suitable products for decontamination
- work surface joins should be sealed to prevent the accumulation of contaminated matter and aid cleaning
- all work surface junctions should be rounded or coved to aid cleaning.

6.12 CHOICE OF EQUIPMENT

When selecting new equipment, you should think about –
- what you want the equipment to do – will the equipment selected be fit for this purpose? Is there any evidence? Is it compatible with other equipment in the surgery?
- how easy it will be to use and maintain – is it CE marked (to demonstrate compliance with Medical Devices Regulations)?

- how easy it is to decontaminate - what are the manufacturer's recommendations? When selecting new hand instruments avoid difficult to clean serrated handles and check that hinges are easy to clean
- can the material covering the dental chair and worksurfaces be cleaned and disinfected regularly without deterioration? Check with the manufacturer
- selecting foot-controlled equipment whenever possible
- training – is it required? Will the manufacturer provide it?

6.13 WATER SUPPLIES

All water lines and air lines should be fitted with anti-retraction valves to help prevent contamination of the lines but these valves cannot be relied upon to prevent infected material being aspirated back into the tubing.

Most dental unit waterlines will harbour biofilm, which acts as a reservoir of microbial contamination and may be a source of known pathogens (Legionella spp, for example). A bottled water system can help to control microbial contamination – disinfectants can be introduced into the water supply to reduce the microbial load. The manufacturer's advice on the type and strength of disinfectant should be followed.

The design of some dental equipment requiring a water supply means that it is possible for contaminated water to be drawn back through the waterlines to the mains water supply (backflow/backsiphonage). Interrupting the water supply to the surgery by a physical break (air gap) will prevent the possibility of backflow. Some equipment requiring a water supply is now manufactured to incorporate an air gap – check this with the manufacturer.

6.14 DECONTAMINATION OF INSTRUMENTS AND EQUIPMENT

All instruments contaminated with oral and other body fluids must be thoroughly cleaned and sterilised after use. Instruments selected for a treatment session but not used must be regarded as contaminated. There are three stages to the decontamination process: pre-sterilisation cleaning, sterilisation, and storage. Manufacturers are now required to provide instructions for the decontamination of their equipment – these instructions should be followed. It is worth checking with the manufacturers prior to purchase that equipment can be used for the purpose intended and decontaminated by the methods used in the practice.

A systematic approach to the decontamination of instruments after use will ensure that dirty instruments are segregated from clean.

6.15   PRE-STERILISATION CLEANING

Used instruments are often heavily contaminated with blood and saliva and must be completely cleaned before sterilisation. Instruments can be cleaned by hand, in an ultrasonic bath or using an instrument washer/disinfector – do check with the manufacturer that instruments can withstand ultrasonic cleaning and automated processing. Ultrasonic cleaners and washer/disinfectors are preferred over hand-cleaning instruments as they are much more effective and contact with contaminated instruments is kept to a minimum thereby reducing the likelihood of inoculation injuries.

After cleaning, all instruments must be examined thoroughly and, if there is residual debris, re-cleaned.

Hand cleaning of dental instruments is the least efficient cleaning method. If this method is used, however, the instruments should be fully immersed in a sink pre-filled with warm water and detergent and a long-handled kitchen-type brush used to remove debris. Instruments should be washed under water with the sharp end of the instrument held away from the body; extra care must be taken when cleaning instruments that are sharp at both ends. Thick waterproof household gloves must be worn to protect against accidental injury and protective eyewear to shield against splashing. The brush used to remove debris from the instruments should be cleaned and autoclaved at regular intervals – at the end of each clinical session, for example. Cleaned brushes should be stored dry.

Ultrasonic cleaners should be used and serviced according to the manufacturer's instructions and should contain a detergent not a disinfectant – disinfectant solutions alone can precipitate proteins and make them resistant to removal. Do check the manufacturer's recommendations. The liquid in the ultrasonic cleaners should be disposed of at the end of each clinical session and more often if it appears heavily contaminated. Ultrasonic cleaners with baskets are preferred. The cleaning cycle should not be interrupted to add further instruments. At the end of each day, the ultrasonic cleaner must be emptied, cleaned and left dry.

Washer/disinfectors designed for cleaning instruments are now available and, if used, the manufacturer's instructions should be followed. Washer/disinfectors are more efficient at pre-sterilisation cleaning than ultrasonic cleaners and hand cleaning, but must not be used as a substitute for sterilisation procedures.

6.16   STERILISATION

The method of choice for the sterilisation of all dental instruments is autoclaving. Sterilisation should be performed at the highest temperature compatible with the instruments in the load. For dental instruments and equipment, autoclaves should reach a temperature of 134–137°C for 3 minutes. New autoclaves should have an integral printer to allow the parameters reached during the sterilisation cycle to be recorded for routine monitoring. Hot air ovens, ultra-violet light, boiling water and chemiclaves are not recommended for sterilising dental instruments and equipment.

Effective sterilisation depends on steam condensing on all surfaces of the instruments in the load to be autoclaved, so it is essential that instruments be placed to allow free circulation of steam; the autoclave chamber must not be overloaded. The sterilisation process is impaired or prevented by air remaining in the chamber or trapped in the load items. Air is removed from the autoclave chamber by either being displaced downwards by steam or by evacuating the air to create a vacuum before steam is introduced into the chamber. For many years, downward displacement autoclaves were the only autoclaves used in a dental surgery; they are still considered an acceptable means of sterilising dental instruments and equipment.

More recently, however, vacuum-phase autoclaves have become available to dentists in general practice. Dentists considering purchasing a vacuum-phase autoclave should ensure that it is capable of sterilising the intended load items (various types are available and not all are suitable for processing dental equipment). The autoclave should be equipped only with cycles providing a pre-sterilisation vacuum stage to minimise the possibility of an incorrect cycle being selected – and a consequent failure to sterilise the load.

Processing wrapped instruments in a conventional downward displacement autoclave may result in inadequate air removal and failure to sterilise. Wrapped instruments and instruments in pouches must be sterilised using a vacuum-phase autoclave.

There continues to be debate about the effective decontamination of handpieces. In theory, a vacuum-phase autoclave will remove the air from the lumen of a dental handpiece, allowing steam to penetrate. The presence of lubricating oil, however, may compromise the sterilisation process. Current opinion is that effective pre-sterilisation cleaning of dental handpieces and subsequent processing in a properly functioning downward displacement autoclave is acceptable.

All autoclaves must be regularly serviced and maintained according to the manufacturer's recommendations and periodically inspected (usually annually) to ensure the integrity of the associated pipework. Vacuum-phase autoclaves are more complicated than conventional steam sterilisers and require more rigorous testing by the user to demonstrate that they function correctly. If you are considering purchasing a vacuum-phase autoclave, you must be aware of all the user tests that you will be required to perform and record on a regular basis. Your service and maintenance agreement should cover the anticipated response time in the event that the autoclave breaks down or malfunctions.

At the end of each day, the residual water should be drained from the auto-clave chamber and reservoir, which should then be cleaned and left open to dry overnight. Many autoclaves now incorporate a facility for draining residual water. A drain valve can be retro-fitted to many autoclaves that do not have an integral drainage device. As a last resort, the high volume suction unit may be used (if it is conveniently placed). If this is necessary, the autoclave should not be moved or lifted unless it can be done safely and without risk of injury.

It is important that the water used in the autoclave should contain no min-erals that may cause damage and, to ensure the integrity of the sterilisation cycle, it should be free of pathogens and endotoxins (pyrogen free).

Successful sterilisation depends upon the consistent reproducibility of sterilising conditions:

- autoclaves must be validated before use and their performance monitored routinely (by periodic testing, including daily and weekly user tests)
- the equipment must be properly maintained according to the manufacturer's instructions
- correct operation of the autoclave must be checked whenever the auto-clave is used by recording the readings (physical parameters) on the auto-clave's instruments or printout at the beginning of each clinical session
- the readings should be compared with the recommended values – if any reading is outside its specified limits, the sterilisation cycle must be regarded as unsatisfactory, irrespective of the results obtained from chemi-cal indicators, and the autoclave cycle checked again. If the second cycle is unsatisfactory, the autoclave should not be used until the problem has been rectified by an engineer
- autoclave logs and printouts should be retained for inspection and monitoring – to demonstrate that the autoclave is performing within the recommended parameters.

Chemical and biological indicators do not demonstrate sterility of the load. Chemical indicators serve only to distinguish loads that have been processed in an autoclave from those that have not. Biological indicators are of limited value in moist heat sterilisation and can only be regarded as additional to the measurement of physical parameters.

Handpieces must be cleaned and autoclaved after each patient. Pre-sterilisation cleaning machines are recommended. Those using an alcohol/disinfectant combination or a washing cycle must only be used to disinfect handpieces on the manufacturer's advice. These machines do not replace the sterilisation process.

6.17 DECONTAMINATION OF HANDPIECES

If a cleaning machine is not used, the following protocol should be adopted for the pre-sterilisation cleaning of handpieces:

- leave the bur in place during cleaning to prevent contamination of the handpiece bearing
- clean the outside of the handpiece with detergent and water – never clean or immerse the handpiece in disinfectant
- remove the bur
- if recommended by the manufacturer, lubricate the handpiece with pressurised oil until clean oil appears out of the chuck and clean off excess oil
- sterilise in an autoclave
- if recommended by the manufacturer, lubricate the handpiece after sterilisation and run it briefly before use to clear excess lubricant
- the oil used for pre-sterilisation cleaning/lubrication should not be the same as used for post-sterilisation lubrication; either two canisters should be used or the nozzle changed between applications.

6.18   INSTRUMENT STORAGE

Sterilised instruments should be stored in dry, covered conditions – trays with lids are now available for this purpose. Sterilised instruments should not be stored in a disinfectant or antiseptic solution. Pouches can be useful for storing infrequently used instruments such as extraction forceps and elevators. Pouches with a clear side allow instruments to be easily identified before opening.

The instruments necessary for treatment should be selected prior to the treatment session. If additional instruments are needed during treatment, care must be taken to avoid the cross contamination of other instruments. Tray systems can help with this.

6.19   SINGLE-USE (DISPOSABLE) ITEMS

Equipment that is described by the manufacturer as 'single use' should be used whenever possible and discarded after use, never reused. 'Single use' means that a device can be used on a patient during one treatment session and then discarded. These items include, but are not limited to, local anaesthetic needles and cartridges, scalpel blades, saliva ejectors, matrix bands, impression trays and beakers. Disposable towels are recommended. Items such as three-in-one tips are difficult to decontaminate effectively and can now be bought as disposable items.

6.20   SURFACE CLEANING AND DISINFECTION

Surfaces of dental units must be impervious as they may become contaminated with potentially infective material. When selecting equipment, consider the ease with which the surfaces can be cleaned and disinfected. Check with the manufacturer that the surfaces are resistant to common disinfectants. The manufacturer may recommend the use of a particular disinfectant; ensure that it will destroy or deactivate all viruses, bacteria and fungi.

Protect light and chair hand controls with disposable impervious coverings and change between patients. If these are not used, the controls must be effectively decontaminated between patients as described below.

A strict system of zoning simplifies the decontamination process. In practice, this means defining the areas, which will become contaminated during operative procedures; only these areas need to be cleaned and disinfected between patients. A surgery can, as a result, be cleaned rapidly. In addition, between clinical sessions, all work surfaces, including those apparently uncontaminated, should be thoroughly cleaned and disinfected.

Effective surface decontamination is a two-stage process of cleaning and disinfection to reduce the microbial load to a minimum
- clear the work surface of instruments, materials, patients' notes etc.
- cleaning is achieved by applying a detergent liquid to the surface and physically wiping the area with a generous application of elbow grease!
- the surface can then be disinfected with a disinfectant that will destroy or deactivate all microbes. Disinfectant solutions must be made up and used according to the manufacturer's instructions
- disinfectants containing alcohol may be flammable and should not be used near a naked flame
- protective gloves must be worn and eyes must be protected
- good general ventilation will help to minimise inhalation.

All aspirators, drains and spittoons should be cleaned after every session with a surfactant/detergent (to break down the biofilm) and a non-foaming disinfectant. Portable aspirators with reservoir bottles are not recommended; they are not fitted with filters and pose a considerable hazard when disposing of the contents.

6.21 DECONTAMINATION OF INSTRUMENTS AND EQUIPMENT PRIOR TO SERVICE OR REPAIR

There is a statutory duty to ensure instruments and equipment are safe for repair. In practice, this means that handpieces and other instruments must be cleaned and sterilised before being sent for repair and a statement confirming this must accompany the equipment. Equipment that cannot be sterilised must be thoroughly cleaned and disinfected in accordance with the manufacturer's instructions.

Decontamination of impression materials and prosthetic and orthodontic appliances.

The responsibility for ensuring impressions and appliances have been cleaned and disinfected prior to dispatch to the laboratory lies solely with the dentist:

- immediately on removal from the mouth, the impression or appliance should be rinsed under running water to remove saliva, blood and debris
- continue the process until it is visibly clean. If an appliance is grossly contaminated, it should be cleaned in an ultrasonic bath containing detergent and then rinsed
- the impression or appliance should be disinfected according to the manufacturer's recommendations. Generic materials such as sodium hypochlorite (household bleach) may no longer be suitable for disinfecting impressions unless specifically recommended by the manufacturer
- disinfectants should not be sprayed onto the surface of the impression; it lessens the effectiveness and creates an inhalation risk. Immersion of the impression is recommended
- the impression or appliance should be rinsed again in water before sending to the laboratory accompanied by a confirmation that it has been disinfected.

Products that are suitable for the disinfection of impressions or appliances are CE marked to demonstrate conformity to European Directives. The manufacturer's recommendations for the dilution of the disinfectant and immersion time must be followed.

6.22 DISPOSAL OF CLINICAL WASTE

All waste in the practice should be segregated into clinical and non-clinical waste –

- clinical waste is waste that is contaminated with blood, saliva or other body fluids and may prove hazardous to any person coming into contact with it
- clinical waste sacks must be no more than three-quarters full, have the air gently squeezed out to avoid bursting when handled by others, labelled and tied at the neck, not knotted
- sharps waste (needles and scalpel blades) must be sealed in UN type approved puncture-proof containers (to BS 7320), which must be labelled before disposal
- local anaesthetic cartridges, whether partially discharged (hazardous) or fully discharged must always be disposed of via the sharps container
- sharps containers should be disposed of when no more than two-thirds full
- clinical waste and sharps waste must be stored securely before collection for final disposal – usually by high-temperature incineration
- clinical waste must only be collected for disposal by a registered waste carrier who holds a certificate of registration

- when waste is collected for disposal, a transfer note must be completed and signed by both parties. The transfer note provides the dentist with evidence that the waste will be disposed of in the correct manner
- repeated transfers of the same kind of waste between the same parties can be covered by one transfer note for up to one year but a copy must be kept for two years.

In some areas there are local arrangements for the collection and disposal of clinical waste; otherwise, arrangements for the collection of clinical waste should be made with a private contractor.

Partially used local anaesthetic cartridges are regarded as hazardous waste and are subject to additional disposal controls; when the waste is collected, consignment notes must be completed and kept for three years. If a local anaesthetic cartridge is fully discharged, however, it is not regarded as hazardous waste and can be disposed of as clinical waste via the sharps container. If partially discharged local anaesthetic cartridges are disposed of via the sharps container, the container must be disposed of as hazardous waste.

Amalgam-filled extracted teeth cannot be discarded via the sharps container, as amalgam must not be incinerated. These teeth should be disposed of with waste amalgam but care should be taken as the teeth will be contaminated with blood. Waste collection agencies often produce special containers for the disposal of amalgam-filled teeth. It is possible to send amalgam-filled teeth (and non-filled teeth) through the post to universities for teaching and research purposes but the patient's consent must be obtained first (and recorded in the clinical records). It is important to ensure that extracted teeth that are sent through the post are first decontaminated and packaged securely to avoid the package being split open during transit. Some dental schools provide a container and disinfectant suitable for decontamination, storage and transport.

A dentist who fails to dispose of waste in a safe manner will face prosecution by the authorities (Environmental Health Departments, Health and Safety Executive etc.) and may be liable to proceedings for serious professional misconduct before the General Dental Council. Clinical waste and hazardous waste must never be disposed of at local refuse tips or landfill sites.

6.23 BLOOD SPILLAGES

If blood is spilled – either from a container or as a result of an operative procedure – the spillage should be dealt with as soon as possible. The spilled blood should be completely covered either by disposable towels, which are then treated with 10 000 ppm sodium hypochlorite solution or by sodium dichloroisocyanurate granules. At least 5 minutes must elapse before the towels etc. are cleared and disposed of as clinical waste. The dental health care worker who deals with the spillage must wear appropriate protective clothing, which will include household gloves, protective eyewear and a disposable apron and, in the case of an extensive floor spillage, protective footwear. Good ventilation is essential.

6.24 BIOPSY SPECIMENS SENT THROUGH THE POST

Dentists using Royal Mail to send patients' non-fixed specimens to pathology laboratories for diagnostic opinion or tests must comply with the UN 602 packaging requirements. The 602 packaging requirements ensure that strict performance tests (including drop and puncture tests) have been met. In practice this means –

- the outer shipping package must bear the UN packaging specification marking. Only first class letter post, special delivery or data post services must be used. The parcel post must not be used
- every pathological specimen must be enclosed in a primary container that is watertight and leakproof
- the primary container must be wrapped in sufficient absorbent material to absorb all fluid in case of breakage
- the primary container should then be protected by placing it in a second durable watertight, leakproof container
- several wrapped primary containers may be placed in one secondary container provided sufficient additional absorbent material is used to cushion the primary containers
- finally the secondary container should be placed in an outer shipping package which protects it and its contents from physical damage and water whilst in transit
- the shipping package must be conspicuously labelled 'PACKED IN COMPLIANCE WITH THE POST OFFICE INLAND LETTER POST SCHEME'
- the sender must also sign and date the package in the space provided
- information concerning the sample, such as data forms, letters and descriptive information should be taped to the outside of the secondary container.

A dentist sending a pathological specimen through the post without complying with the above requirements may be liable to prosecution.

Specimens that are 'fixed' are not covered by these requirements. This means that –

- specimens should be enclosed in a primary container and sealed securely
- the container must be wrapped in sufficient absorbent material to absorb all leakage if it is damaged, and then sealed in a leakproof plastic bag
- the specimen should then be placed in a padded bag and labelled 'PATHOLOGICAL SPECIMEN – FRAGILE WITH CARE'

- the bag must show the name and address of the sender to be contacted in case of damage or leakage.

6.25 PERSONAL PROTECTION

The employing dentist has a duty of care towards employees to provide a safe place of work. It is not sufficient simply to provide personal protective equipment such as gloves and glasses; the employer must ensure that it is being used in the correct manner. It is important that all staff understand the principles of personal protection and that compliance is part of their contracts of employment.

6.26 IMMUNISATION

All clinical staff should be vaccinated against the common illnesses. All those involved in clinical procedures must be vaccinated against hepatitis B. If an inoculation injury is sustained before completion of the course, follow-up action, including boosters and tests for hepatitis B markers, is essential. The hepatitis B vaccine is effective in preventing infection in individuals who produce specific antibodies to the hepatitis B surface antigen (anti-HBs). UK experts recommend that anti-HBs level of >100 mIU/ml will provide protection against hepatitis B infection.

It is now clear that immunological memory is produced in those who respond to the primary course of the vaccine (>100 mIU/ml). Protection against infection is maintained even if antibody concentrations at the time of exposure have declined.

Anti-HBs levels must be measured 2–4 months after completion of the immunisation course.

A single booster dose five years after completion of the primary course is recommended for all health care workers who have contact with blood, blood-stained fluids and patients' tissues. Pre- and post-testing at the time of a booster is not required if the individual responded to the primary course of the vaccine.

Not everyone will respond to the vaccine, however, some because they are true non-responders, others because they carry the virus. Those who fail to respond should undergo further investigation to establish if test markers of hepatitis B infection are present. Investigation to establish infection should take place before booster doses of the vaccine are given in an attempt to achieve anti-HBs levels of at least 100 mIU/ml.

True vaccine non-responders may remain susceptible to infection and it is essential that inoculation injuries be followed up with tests for hepatitis B markers where appropriate.

Dental clinicians and their staff must have documentary evidence to demonstrate that they have been immunised and their response to the vaccine checked. Where they have failed to respond they must undergo further investigation to exclude the possibility of being high risk carriers of the hepatitis B virus. The employing dentists must hold evidence of hepatitis B immunisation; post-vaccination blood test results will show whether an adequate level of immunity has been achieved. The letter (left) may be helpful, if you are requesting this information from your employee's general medical practitioner. Do remember that you must have the consent of your employee before you approach his/her GMP and that any information provided is confidential and should be stored appropriately.

Hepatitis B infection in pregnant women may result in severe disease for the mother and chronic infection in the newborn. Although infants can receive active/passive immunisation at birth, vaccination should not be withheld from a pregnant woman if she is likely to be at risk from contracting hepatitis B infection. Many women have discovered at a later date that, at the time of receiving the vaccine, they were pregnant. In these instances, the vaccine caused no harm to themselves or their children. The vaccine also does not affect fertility and does not prevent breast-feeding.

6.27 HAND PROTECTION

The care of hands is vital to infection control; lacerated, abraded and cracked skin can offer a portal of entry for micro-organisms. Gloves must be worn for all clinical procedures and treated as single-use items so a new pair of gloves must be used for each patient. Gloves should be donned immediately before contact with the patient and removed as soon as clinical treatment is complete. Used gloves must be disposed of as clinical waste.

Recommendations for hand care during clinical sessions include –
- removal of rings, jewellery and watches
- covering all cuts and abrasions with waterproof adhesive dressings
- methodical handwashing using a good quality liquid soap preferably containing a disinfectant – a full handwash and thorough drying is recommended before donning gloves
- removing gloves and washing hands after each patient (gives the hands time to recover from being covered)
- regular use of an emollient hand cream to prevent the skin from drying, especially after every clinical session.

There is a variety of gloves available. Those selected should be –
- good quality non-sterile medical gloves (to European standard BSEN 455, parts 1 and 2, medical gloves for single use), worn for all clinical procedures and changed after every patient

- well fitting and non-powdered. The powder from gloves can contaminate veneers and radiographs, disperse allergenic proteins into the surgery atmosphere and interfere with wound healing
- 'hypoallergenic' and 'low protein' to reduce the possibility of allergy.

Allergic contact dermatitis is rare but, if it develops, it may be serious enough to cause the person to cease practice. If it is suspected, the advice of a dermatologist should be sought. Irritant contact dermatitis is more common and can be avoided by careful choice of glove and hand disinfectant and meticulous hand care.

Increasingly, dentists are encountering patients who are allergic to latex or the chemicals used in glove manufacture. Non-latex gloves are available but additional precautions will be needed to protect the allergic patient against contact with latex through other sources in the surgery – local anaesthetic cartridges, rubber dam and protective glasses, for example. A Fact File on Hand dermatitis and latex allergy is available from the BDA. The advice of a consultant immunologist may need to be sought on the treatment of the patient.

6.28 EYE PROTECTION AND FACE MASKS

Operators and close support clinical staff must protect their eyes against foreign bodies, splatter and aerosols that may arise during operative dentistry, especially during scaling (manual and ultrasonic), the use of rotary instruments, cutting and use of wires and the cleaning of instruments. Ideally, protective glasses should have side protection. Many modern prescription glasses have small lenses, which would make them unsuitable for use as eye protection. Patients' eyes must always be protected against possible injury; tinted glasses may also protect against glare from the operating light.

Masks do not confer complete microbiological protection but they do stop splatter from contaminating the face. Masks or visors are recommended for all operative procedures and should be changed after every patient, not pulled down or re-used.

6.29 SURGERY CLOTHING

A wide variety of clothing is worn in dental surgeries and in many practices is used to reinforce the corporate image. There is no consensus view on whether surgery clothing should have short or long sleeves. Short sleeves will allow the forearms to be washed as part of the handwashing routine. Long-sleeved coats or tunics will protect the skin of the arms against splatter. This is important if skin is cracked or abraded (as a result of eczema, for example). Long sleeves, however, are more likely to become contaminated during clinical sessions and could cause a breach in infection control. Surgery clothing should be made of a material that can be machine-washed with a suitable detergent at a temperature of 65°C to eradicate any potential microbial contamination.

6.30 AEROSOL AND SALIVA/BLOOD SPLATTER

Good surgery ventilation and efficient high-volume aspirators, which exhaust externally from the premises, will reduce the risk of infection by dispersing and eliminating aerosols. External vents should discharge without risk to the public or re-circulation into any building. Aspirators and tubing should be cleaned and disinfected regularly in accordance with the manufacturer's instructions and the system should be flushed through at the end of each session with their recommended surfactant/detergent and/or non-foaming disinfecting agent.

Rubber dam isolation of teeth also offers substantial advantages and should be used whenever practicable. It enhances the quality of the operative environment and virtually abolishes saliva/blood splatter and aerosols. When working without rubber dam, the use of high-volume aspiration is essential.

6.31 INOCULATION INJURIES

Inoculation injuries are the most likely route for transmission of blood-borne viral infections in dentistry. The definition of an inoculation injury includes all incidents where a contaminated object or substance breaches the integrity of the skin or mucous membranes or comes into contact with the eyes. The following are typical examples
- sticking or stabbing with a used needle or other instrument
- splashes with a contaminated substance to the eye or other open lesion
- cuts with contaminated equipment
- bites or scratches inflicted by patients.
  Inoculation injuries must be dealt with promptly and correctly –
- the wound should be allowed to bleed and washed thoroughly with running water
- where there is reason to be concerned about the possible transmission of infection, the injured person should seek urgent advice according to the local arrangements in place on what follow-up action, including serological surveillance, is necessary. Ideally all practices should have formal links with an occupational health service, so that management of sharps injuries is undertaken promptly and according to accepted national protocols

- every primary care trust will have at least one designated specialist, for example the Consultant in Communicable Disease Control or Consultant Medical Microbiology, who can be contacted for advice on post-exposure prophylaxis (PEP). Every practice should have details of the local contact displayed prominently
- when local advice cannot be obtained, advice should be obtained from the following sources

England: the duty doctor at the PHLS Communicable Disease Surveillance Centre, 61 Colindale Avenue, London NW9 5EQ (Tel: 020 8200 6868)

Scotland: Scottish Centre for Infection and Environmental Health (SCIEH), Clifton House, Clifton Place, Glasgow G3 7LN (Tel: 0141 300 1100)

Wales: PHL Cardiff, The University Hospital of Wales, Heath Park, Cardiff CF14 4XW (Tel: 02920 742718)

Northern Ireland: Director of Public Health at your local Health and Social Services Board

- a full record of the incident should be made in the accident book and include details of who was injured, how the incident occurred, what action was taken, which dentists were informed and when and, if known, the name of the patient being treated. Both the injured person and the dentist in charge should countersign the record.

The risk of acquiring HIV infection following an inoculation injury is small. If the injury is risk-assessed as significant for transmission of HIV (see Table 1.7) and the source patient is HIV infected, the use of anti-retroviral drugs taken prophylactically as soon as possible after exposure – ideally within one hour – is recommended. Post-exposure prophylaxis involves the use of a short course (4 weeks) of treatment with anti-retroviral drugs in an attempt to reduce even further the risk of infection with HIV following exposure. Dentists should clarify local arrangements for urgent access to PEP, with the help of an occupational health department or a consultant in communicable diseases, before any incident occurs.

6.32   INFECTION CONTROL POLICY

Each practice must have a written infection control policy. The policy should describe the practice policy for all aspects of infection control and provide a useful guide to the training necessary for each member of staff to be competent and confident in its implementation. All members of the dental team must know who is responsible for ensuring certain activities are carried out and whom to report any accidents or incidents. Accidents and incidents should always be recorded in the accident book. Some accidents and incidents must be reported to the Health and Safety Executive; for further information on this see the BDA's advice sheet on Health and Safety Law for Dental

Practice (A3). Accidents and incidents involving the failure of dental instruments or equipment should be reported to the MDA.

Although a policy will describe the procedure for the practice as a whole, it is useful for each member of staff to receive a copy and to sign a declaration to confirm that the policy has been received and training provided – for example, 'I confirm that I have read the practice Infection Control Policy and have received training in all its aspects'. A copy of the policy should be displayed in each surgery (Table 1.7).

It is a good idea to discuss infection control at practice staff meetings. Open discussion will allow misunderstandings to be addressed and ensure that everyone in the practice approaches infection control in the same way.

You might not be the only person who is unclear and it is useful to discuss the policy frequently to ensure that we all understand its implications. Remember, any of our patients might ask you about the policy, so make sure you understand it.

1 All staff must be immunised against hepatitis B and a record of their hepatitis B seroconversion held by the practice owner. For those who do not seroconvert or cannot be immunised medical advice and counselling will be sought. In these cases it may be necessary to restrict their clinical activities.

2 The practice provides protective clothing, gloves, eyewear and masks that must be worn by dentists and PCDs during all operative procedures. Protective clothing worn in the surgery should not be worn outside the practice premises.

3 Before donning gloves, hands must be washed using .... Any glove that becomes damaged must be replaced and a new pair of gloves must be used for each patient.

4 Before sterilisation, re-usable instruments should be cleaned either by placing in the ultrasonic cleaner or washer/disinfector or washed in a designated area by hand under water using a long-handled brush. Inspect instruments for residual debris and re-clean if necessary. Instruments are then rinsed under running water before being sterilised using

---

Table 1.7 An example of a practice infection control policy for display

Infection control is of prime importance in this practice. It is essential to the safety of our patients, our families and us. Every member of staff will receive training in all aspects of infection control, including decontamination of dental instruments and equipment, and the following policy must be adhered to at all times. If there is any aspect that is not clear, please ask ....

an autoclave. Heavy-duty gloves and eye protection must be worn when handling and cleaning used instruments. All instruments that have been potentially contaminated must be sterilised. Single-use items must not be decontaminated and re-used.

5 Sterilised instruments should be stored in covered trays/pouches.

6 Working areas that have instruments placed on them during treatment will be kept to a minimum, clearly identified and, after each patient, cleaned with .... (detergent) and disinfected using ....

7 Needles should be re-sheathed only using the re-sheathing device provided. Needles, scalpel blades, LA cartridges, burs, matrix bands etc. shall be disposed of in the yellow sharps container. This must never be more than two-thirds full.

8 All clinical waste must be placed in the appropriate sacks or bins provided in each surgery. The sack must be securely fastened when three-quarters full and stored in the designated area.

9 All dental impressions must be rinsed until visibly clean and disinfected using .... (as recommended by the manufacturer) and labelled as 'disinfected' before being sent to the laboratory. Technical work being returned to the laboratory should also be disinfected and labelled.

10 In the event of an inoculation injury, the wound should be allowed to bleed, washed thoroughly under running water and covered with a waterproof dressing. The incident should be immediately discussed with .... to assess whether further action is needed. Advice on post-exposure prophylaxis can be obtained from.................................... Record the incident in the accident book.

11 Any spillages involving blood or saliva or mercury will be reported to ....

12 Anyone developing a reaction to protective gloves or a chemical must inform .... immediately.

13 ALL STAFF WILL OBSERVE TOTAL CONFIDENTIALITY OF ALL INFORMATION RELATING TO PATIENTS OF THE PRACTICE

Date........................Review date.......................

6.33 INFECTION CONTROL CHECKLIST

At start of day/session

- Fill the autoclave reservoir and run the autoclave for a complete cycle
- Record the sterilisation parameters reached in your autoclave logbook
- Compare these with the manufacturer's recommended parameters

Before patient treatment

- Ensure that all equipment has been sterilised or adequately disinfected (if it cannot be sterilised)
- Put disposable coverings in place where necessary
- Place only the appropriate instruments on bracket table
- Set out all materials and other essential instruments
- Update patient's medical history

During patient treatment

- Treat all patients as potentially infectious
- Wear gloves, masks and protective eyewear and protective clothing
- Provide eye protection for patient
- Wash hands before gloving; a new pair of gloves must be used for each patient
- Change gloves immediately if they are torn, cut or punctured
- Use rubber dam to isolate where appropriate
- Use high-volume aspiration
- Ensure good general ventilation of the treatment area
- Handle sharps carefully and only re-sheath needles using a suitable device

After patient treatment

- Dispose of sharps via the sharps container
- Segregate and dispose of clinical waste
- Clean and inspect all instruments to ensure visibly clean before placing in an ultrasonic cleaning machine or washer/disinfector
- Sterilise cleaned instruments using an autoclave and store covered
- Clean and disinfect all contaminated work surfaces
- Clean and disinfect impressions and other dental appliances before sending to laboratory
- Prepare surgery for next patient

At the end of each session

- Dispose of all clinical waste from the surgery area
- Clean and disinfect all work surfaces thoroughly
- Disinfect the aspirator, its tubing and the spittoon
- Clean the chair and the unit
- Empty and clean ultrasonic cleaning machine and leave to dry.

At the end of the day

- Drain autoclave chamber and water reservoir to remove all residual water and leave to dry

REFERENCES

Carson P, Freeman R. Tell-show-do: reducing anticipatory anxiety an emergency paediatric Dental Patients. *International Journal of Health Promotion and Education* 1998; 36:87–90.

Freeman R, Adams EK, Gelbier S. The provision of primary dental care for patients with special needs. *Primary Dental Care* 1997;4:31–34.

Freeman R, Carson P. Relative analgesia and general dental practitioners: attitudes and intentions to provide conscious sedation for paediatric dental extractions. *International Journal of Paediatric Dentistry* 2003;13:320–326.

General Dental Council. *Maintaining Standards: Guidance to Dentists on Professional and Personal Conduct.* London, GDC, 1997.

Ibbetson R. Choosing a career in dentistry. *Dent Update* 2003;30:28–36.

Kelly M, Steele J, Nuttall N, Bradnock G. Morris J *et al.,* Adult Dental Health. *Surrey survey* 1998, London HMSO.

Laing and Buisson. (2003) UK DENTAL CARE–Market Sector Report. CIGNA.

Scott BJJ. So you want to be an academic? *Dent Update* 2003;30:in press.

Survey Oral Health in the United Kingdom 1988. London, 2000, The Stationery Office.

Willumsen T, Vassend O, Hoffart A. One-year follow-up for the dental fear: effects of cognitice therapy, applied relation and nitrous oxide sedation. *Acta Odontol Scand* 2001; 59:335–340.

2 Practice building – relationships around the patient

1.0 THE DENTIST–PATIENT RELATIONSHIP

Patients' satisfaction with their dentist and the dental health care they receive is critical not only in the choice of practice but also with regard to their loyalty to the practice. The need for patients to be able to accept the treatment that the dentist offers and to return for continuous dental care is essential as it allows patients to achieve their dental health goals and provides the dentist with his income and livelihood. The patient should, therefore, be the centre of attention with the dentist's ability to provide acceptable and accessible care pivotal. Goold *et al.* (1999) have stated that the interaction with the patient:

> 'remains the keystone to care … [*it provides*] the medium in which [*informa-tion*] is gathered, diagnoses and plans are made, compliance is accomplished … and support … provided'.

Despite the acknowledgement of the need for understanding and the pro-vision of appropriate health care, recent research has shown that a 'gap' exists between the treatment actions of the dentist and the treatment wishes of the patient (Newsome *et al.* 2000). The 'gap' is exacerbated by the dentist's apparent lack of effective communication skills which is further compounded by his/her use of technical terms and jargon. Rather than being the centre of attention, some patients, according to Newsome *et al.* (2000), feel that they are relegated to the periphery with their treatment wishes remaining unfulfilled.

Although the importance of the dentist–patient interaction has been accepted, difficulties surround its definition and characteristic qualities. This has been a consequence of changes in patients' perceptions of desired care as well as the need for informed consent. The dentist–patient interaction can no longer be envisaged as one person working upon another (the paternalistic model) but rather a two-person endeavour characterised by shared decision-making (the psychodynamic model).

As the ultimate goal of the dentist–patient interaction is joint decision-making, the dentist's ability to communicate effectively with patients is essential. The dentist needs to be able to use his/her communication skills to gather infor-mation, develop and maintain a therapeutic relationship (treatment alliance) and provide information to patients in a manner in which they can understand to enable patients to make informed choice. A new type of dentist–patient relationship has gradually emerged. It is characterised by (Freeman 2000):
1. its dynamic quality,
2. the equality of the health professional–patient interaction; and
3. the ability of both parties to participate in a joint decision-making.

Within this environment patients tend to be more compliant and partici-pate with preventive advice, experience greater quality of life and higher satis-faction with the health care provided (Goold *et al.* 1999). It seems that those patients who are made to feel welcomed are listened to and are encouraged to participate in their treatment decisions, are those who express greater satisfaction and remain loyal to the general practice.

If such patient management goals are to be achieved then dentists must be proficient in their knowledge and skills in this regard. In order that this may be accomplished it is necessary to recognise factors which enable or inhibit the formation of the treatment relationship between the dentist and his/her patient, to dissect the dentist–patient interaction into its constituent parts and to examine the structural elements of the dental interview.

1.1 FACTORS ENABLING THE INFORMATION OF THE DENTIST–PATIENT RELATIONSHIP

Factors which enable the formation and maintenance of the dentist–patient relationship belong with both participants – the dentist and the patient. In many respects the psycho-social influences which affect the dentist are similar to those that concern the patient. The ability of the dentist to communicate effectively by actively listening to the patient's words are mirrored by the patient's ability to be able to speak freely and to divulge worries, concerns and anxieties.

The dentist's understanding of the dentist–patient relationship and the need to provide empathy is reflected in the patient's trust that their words and views will be acceptable to the practitioner. It is clear that in order to have an awareness of factors which influence the formation and maintenance of the dentist–patient relationship it is necessary to consider factors which influence both the dentist and patient (fig. 2.1).

1.2 UNDERSTANDING THE DENTIST–PATIENT RELATIONSHIP: THE TREATMENT ALLIANCE

Various models have been proposed to explain the clinician–patient relationship. These have included early ideas which considered the relationship with the patient as a dynamic continuum from active (dentist)–passive (patient) to guidance (dentist)–participation (patient) (Szaz and Hollander 1956). New models have replaced earlier concepts (Falkum and Førde 2001) and have the tendency to be more static than dynamic, explaining only one aspect of the relationship with the clinician. The new explanatory models include the paternalistic model, the consumer model, the interpretative model, the deliberative model and the negotiation model. Using these models it was hoped that a way forward could be envisaged in which concerns about the 'asymmetrical and imbalanced' relationship with the patient could be addressed.

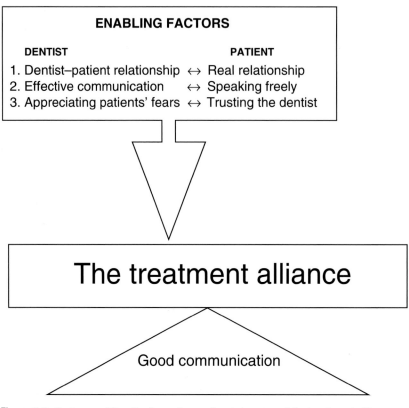

Figure 2.1 Factors enabling the formation and maintenance of the treatment alliance.

The asymmetry of the relationship between the patient and the health professional has been related to the patient complying with the dentist's treatment decisions. In what has been described as a paternalistic model the dentist presents the patient with a series of treatment options from which s/he informs the patient of the option s/he feels will restore the patient's dental health and/or reduce pain. Difficulties inherent within this model are associated with the idea that the dentist 'knows what is best' and disregards the patient's treatment wishes.

At the other extreme is the 'consumer model'. Whereas in the paternalistic model the dentist dictated; in the consumer model, the patient is autonomous. The dentist acts only as a provider of information – his/her views and opinions are unimportant – it is the independent patient who decides on treatment.

The interpretative model

The interpretative model combines aspects of the paternalistic and consumer models. The dentist acts as the patient's adviser, providing information as to the treatment of choice. The patient is encouraged to speak freely, to voice his/her wishes, worries and anxieties. Together clinician and patient come to a joint decision. However, concerns have been raised as to health professionals' ability to communicate and counsel the patient and the tendency for the interpretative model to be replaced by the paternalistic model.

The advisory model

The advisory, or what is known as the deliberative model, is perceived as the path to joint decision-making (Falkum and Førde 2001). This model embodies the ideal of patient autonomy, the caring physician who counsels rather than imposes, who acknowledges the consequence of his/her own values upon the decision-making process and realises the importance of health-related issues. Despite the apparent dynamic quality of this model it does not provide the health professional with an understanding that the patient's relationship with the clinician changes not only with time but also with the reason for attendance and treatment.

The psychodynamic model

A model, which appreciates the active quality of the dentist and patient interaction, is the psychodynamic model (fig. 2.2). In this the dentist and patient are equally autonomous, negotiating a way forward, sharing information and coming to a joint decision. The psychodynamic model allows for flexibility within the interaction by acknowledging that the patient's relationship status with the dentist does not remain static but changes with time of acquaintance and during treatment (Freeman 2000). There are three elements to the psychodynamic model, which illustrate the changing roles for both participants. These are the real relationship, the treatment alliance, the transference and regression (Greenson 1967).

The real relationship

As the patient enters the surgery the interaction will be primarily based on the patient's recognition of the qualities the dentist possesses in terms of his/her clinical skills (the real relationship). This is very much a reality relationship. The patient has heard of the dentist's patient management and technical skills and as a result has made the decision to choose the practice. The real relationship is an adult-to-adult interaction.

The treatment alliance

The ability of the patient to accept the treatment being offered and provided by the dentist is an expression of the treatment alliance. By acknowledging the importance and equality (adult-to-adult interaction) of the treatment

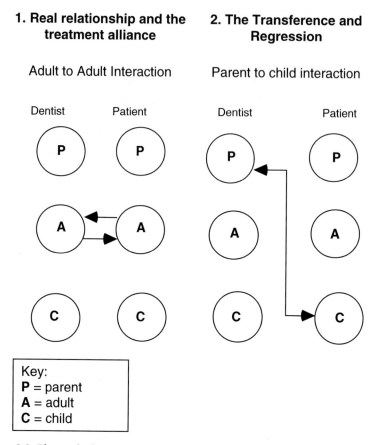

1. Real relationship and the treatment alliance

Adult to Adult Interaction

2. The Transference and Regression

Parent to child interaction

Key:
P = parent
A = adult
C = child

Figure 2.2 The psychodynamic model of the dentist–patient relationship.

alliance provides the dentist with the means of understanding why the patient may be unable to accept the care which is being offered and provided. Kulich *et al.* (2001) have revisited and redefined the concept of the treatment alliance in terms of the dentist's 'relatedness'. Relatedness in this context refers to the ability of the dentist 'to reach, encourage and influence the patient'.

Irrespective of definition the treatment alliance may be considered as the kernel, the very essence of the dentist–patient relationship with the dentist doing everything to nurture and maintain a working relationship or treatment alliance with the patient. It is a consequence of the treatment alliance that the patient can accept the care the dentist provides even in the most adverse circumstances. The creation, nurturing and maintenance of the treatment alliance is founded upon the ability of dental health professionals to communicate effectively with their patients (Freeman 2000, Kulich *et al.* 2000).

The transference and regression

As the chair goes back and treatment begins a change occurs in the interaction between the participants. A transference occurs in which the patient's feelings from the past are transferred and relived, so to speak, in the here and now. The transference is no longer a relationship between adults but one in which the dentist is powerful (as parent) and the patient powerless (as child). The patient may start to perceive the dentist as a caring parent and start to feel like the child they once were. The accompanying change from more controlled to less controlled emotional state is known as regression. This is a temporal state of affair as when the treatment finishes and the chair goes up the relationship between dentist and patient returns to an adult-to-adult interaction.

Which of the above models provides the best understanding of the dentist–patient interaction? The advisory or deliberative model is said to promote the basis for optimal interacting between clinician and patient. However, it only represents one aspect of the dynamic relationship with the patient. When an adult or child patient presents in pain the most appropriate model is the paternalistic model. In other circumstances the patients' need to choose which is the most appropriate form of treatment occurs in situations where costs are an issue. The choice between a partial denture and a bridge belongs with the patient and not the dentist, who in this situation acts as source of information (consumer model). Dental health education interactions with the patient, using motivational interviewing techniques to advise and counsel, are examples of both interpretative and deliberative models.

Perhaps it is better not to think of one model of the dentist–patient relationship but to think of many which can be incorporated into an overarching understanding of the interaction. The psychodynamic model allows each of the above models (paternalistic, consumer, interpretative and deliberative models) to be slotted in and to explain the quality of the various and differing interactions with the patient. The psychodynamic model provides a platform, from which the importance of the treatment alliance as the cornerstone of the dentist–patient relationship can be realised.

It is the maintenance of the treatment alliance in the face of adversity – costs of dental care, oral/dental pain, dental anxiety/phobia and the tendency for regression – which must be sustained for a successful interaction with the patient. Dentists can preserve the treatment alliance by acknowledging the need to walk a tight rope between objectivity on the one hand and empathy on the other. This reflects their acceptance of the role of interpersonal skills in forging the treatment alliance. Using effective communication skills dentists can counteract the effects of the barriers to accepting dental care and establish 'an empathetic milieu' (Massé and Légaré 2001). The treatment alliance between dentist and patient will be strengthened, maintained and preserved and the patient can now accept the mutually agreed treatment that is being offered and provided by the dentist.

1.3 EFFECTIVE COMMUNICATION AND FORGING THE TREATMENT ALLIANCE

The tensions and strains that arise from the initial clinical encounter may put the greatest strain upon the developing treatment alliance. The need to establish an empathetic atmosphere or milieu to foster the treatment alliance can only be achieved by the confident use of the dentist's interpersonal and communication skills.

The negotiation model allows the culture of the dentist (as a health professional) and patient (as a lay person) to be acknowledged as complimentary factors in the development of the treatment alliance. According to Massé and Légaré (2001) for the treatment alliance to be forged the initial meeting with the patient must follow a process, composed of six individual steps:

- Step 1   the establishment of empathy
- Step 2   the dentist communicating effectively
- Step 3   the patient encouraged to openly and freely
- Step 4   the dentist appreciating the patient's fears
- Step 5   the patient trusting the dentist and building rapport
- Step 6   joint decision-making

When this process is finished the successful clinical outcome will be a negotiated treatment plan which is a reflection of the treatment alliance and joint decision-making.

Step 1: The establishment of empathy

The establishment of empathy is the first step in development of the treatment alliance. In order to promote an empathetic atmosphere the dentist must provide a suitable setting, s/he must understand the patient's emotional reactions and restore the patient's role in treatment discussions.

The setting paves the way for success. The dental surgery, however, may have frightening connotations and could be considered a somewhat hostile environment for the establishment of empathy. Furthermore, the routines in the dental surgery may not allow for enough time for the consultation, and tensions may be set up as a consequence of misunderstandings between the dentist and patient.

An awareness of the need to counteract distortions in the communication process and the potential for anxiety, tension and conflict allows the dentist to reconsider the appropriateness of the first clinical encounter occurring in the dental chair. Many dental surgeries have a room set aside to conduct the interviews with new patients. This allows not only for a physical empathetic milieu but also for the real relationship to be maintained. The face-to-face interaction provides the basis for reality-based discussions on such issues as proposed treatment plans, the costs of treatment and treatment outcomes.

The allocated time spent with the patient at the initial clinical encounter is well spent. It is during this time the treatment alliance is forged and the dentist starts to discover more about the patient – oral health beliefs, preventive regimes (diet, oral hygiene, habits), dental anxiety status and details about work and lifestyle.

Steps 2 and 3: Communicating effectively and encouraging the patient to speak

In steps 2 and 3 it is the dentist's ability to communicate effectively with the patient and for the patient to speak freely that allows empathy to be incorporated into the developing treatment alliance.

Communication is a two-way process which reflects the essence of the treatment alliance (two people working together in a joint endeavour) and is essential for the incorporation of empathy to strengthen the dentist–patient interaction. In general there are six key elements in communication. These are

- understanding non-verbal communication,
- listening,
- encouraging people to talk,
- asking questions and obtaining feedback,
- accepting other people's feelings and giving feedback.

The dentist must be able to apply communication and interpersonal skills in a manner which is appropriate and suitable with regard to the type of clinical encounter. How long the dentist has known the patient, the patient's age, oral health beliefs, dental anxiety status, dental treatment experiences and degree of understanding will dictate the type and format of the interaction with the dentist. The skills and techniques appropriate for continuing care are not suitable for an initial clinical encounter and the dentist must dissect the interview into a beginning, middle and end using the communication styles appropriate for each part of the interaction.

Beginning of the interview
From the outset the dentist must encourage the patient to talk in order to establish rapport. It is important that the dentist recognises the significance of both non-verbal and verbal communications in this regard.

The ability of the dentist to listen actively is crucial. Listening involves being aware of all non-verbal cues and acts as a bridge between verbal and non-verbal communications. This is not the usual type of hearing but is a conscious and determined effort to listen to what is being said and what has been omitted. Listening for what is excluded has been described as listening with the 'third ear'. The patient's omissions may reflect his/her fears of the dentist's reactions to critical thoughts, worries resulting from previous dental treatment experiences or concerns about the costs of care.

Non-verbal communications to consider at this stage include:
- eye contact,
- awareness of the patient's body language,
- the speed, pitch, tone, and the way (number of filled pauses) by which the patient is communicating.

Non-verbal cues will provide the dentist with clues as to the patient's thoughts, worries and anxieties with regard to dental treatment. It is beneficial therefore that the dentist maintains eye contact and that the interview takes place in an environment which will allow the dentist to listen carefully to the patient's words and utterances.

At this point in the interview the patient may be unable to speak freely or openly. The dentist who recognises this situation will gently confront the patient using an open question format enabling and encouraging the patient to speak. Open questions are 'beginning questions' and are used to find out more about the patient – his/her oral health beliefs, treatment experiences, needs, wants, feelings and so forth. They encourage the patient to set the agenda and for the dentist to follow, monitoring the patient's answers and responses.

Different types of question (question format) exist and are used at different times (for example, open questions at the start of the interview) and for different purposes (for example, closed questions are used late in the interview to clarify) throughout the interview (Table 2.1).

During the interview
Monitoring the interview by active listening, the dentist can now use focus questions to encourage and support the patient to speak freely. Focused questions are a means of maintaining the momentum of the interview and can

---

Table 2.1 Types, purpose and use of questions

QUESTION:- FORMAT	OPEN	↔	FOCUSED	→	CLOSED
WHEN USED IN THE INTERVIEW	BEGINNING	→	MIDDLE	→	END
PURPOSE OF THE QUESTION	INFORMATION GATHERING (Facilitating)	↔	EXPLAINING + NEGOTIATING (Guiding)	→	YES/NO ANSWERS (clarifying)

GUIDELINES FOR QUESTIONING:
The guidelines include, taking time to think, moving between open, focused and then closed questions during the interview, asking one question at a time, check that the patient has understood what is being asked and *avoiding* leading questions.

be thought of as guiding questions. The patient's responses will help clarify issues raised in the earlier part of the interview. The dentist now has the opportunity to provide explanations and give advice in reply to the patient's concerns. It is important that the dentist's answers are short, concise and jargon-free with key points being highlighted and repeated as necessary.

Ending the interview
The interview ends with closed questioning. Closed questions are a final means of clarifying important points and issues raised by the patient. At this time the dentist can ensure that the patient has understood what has been discussed and this paves the way for joint decision-making.

Step 4: Appreciating the patient's fears

The dentist must not convince the patient but, rather, advise and discuss the treatment options with him/her. In order to do this the dentist has to shift in his/her interacting style. The dentist must allow change to occur and permit the interaction to be 'patient-centred' rather than 'clinician-centred'. The change from 'clinician-centred' to 'patient-centred' is associated with a shift in the dentist's degree of control (fig. 2.3).

With the ever-increasing shifts from instructing to discussing the dentist starts to understand the proposed treatment from the patient's perspective. The patient may have fears, worries and anxieties about the treatment which may be associated with the cost of the treatment, the outcome of the treatment and/or dental anxiety arising from previous treatment experiences.

Armed with this information the dentist is now is a position to present the patient with a treatment plan (Chapter 4) which reflects the patient's perceptions, acknowledges the patient's wishes and ability to tolerate restorative treatment. The negotiated treatment plan also acknowledges the dentist's clinical expertise and his/her ability to withstand the patient's dental anxiety during treatment. In this way a treatment plan is constructed between the

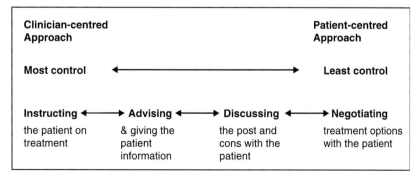

Figure 2.3 Continuum from clinician-centred to patient-centred approaches.

dentist and patient that accepts the wishes of the patient with respect to the clinical needs as diagnosed by the dentist.

Step 5: Trusting the dentist: building rapport

The patient will have been encouraged to speak freely and to voice concerns, worries and anxieties. The dentist's non-judgemental stance will convey to the patient that rapport has been established between them. There are three elements to rapport that reflects a trust element in the interaction with the health professional. These are:
- harmony,
- compatibility, and
- affinity.

The fact that the patient feels a sense of trust means that a change has occurred in the patient's opinion of the dentist. The patient's worries and fears have evaporated. The expected change in the patient's emotional state and a change in the relationship status have not occurred (fig. 2.2) and the dentist is no longer seen as a fearful or frightening parental figure (transference), but a person who is willing to listen, provide explanations and discuss treatment options (fig. 2.2). The dentist, by adopting an expectant attitude, has enabled the patient to voice certain topics, which might on other occasions be difficult to speak about. The dentist's communications have provided a bridge to allow the patient to develop trust in the dentist's treatment decisions.

The patient's trust has allowed a shift to occur and with it the incorporation of some of the dentist's professional opinions. The patient starts to appreciate the dentist's clinical expertise and his/her reasons for the decision of an immediate partial denture rather than a bridge and/or may recognise the importance of home care in the maintenance of his oral health. With the development of trust in the dentist's clinical expertise the patient is ready to consider the proposed treatment offered by the dentist.

Step 6: Joint decision-making

As the interview draws to a close the dentist and patient have come to an accommodation. The dentist has come to understand the patient's beliefs, concerns and anxieties while the patient has come to acknowledge the dentist's clinical skills and expertise. The dentist's ability to encourage the patient's participation in the treatment decision-making has been an important step and together they have negotiated a mutually agreed treatment plan. A plan, which has incorporated professional and lay opinions, values and concerns about treatment, costs, treatment outcome and prognosis.

The use of a patient-centred strategy has allowed the treatment alliance to develop. However, this is merely the first phase in a long process. The treatment

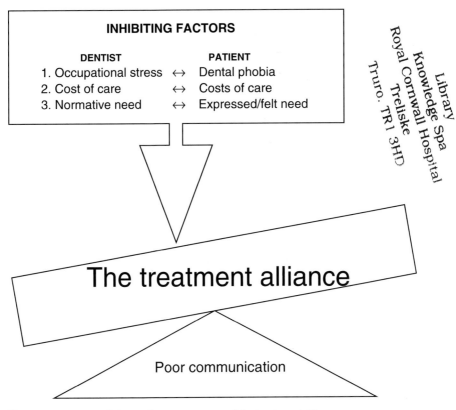

Figure 2.4 Factors inhibiting the maintenance of the treatment alliance.

alliance will become strengthened as the patient's trust and his apprecia-tion of the dentist's skills becomes consolidated. The dentist's awareness of the patient's health care needs will gradually grow and will ensure that the treatment alliance and the dentist–patient relationship take on the mantle of a two-person endeavour. The patient is now able to receive the treatment that the dentist is offering and providing – the treatment alliance has now come of age.

1.4 FACTORS INHIBITING THE FORMATION OF THE DENTIST–PATIENT RELATIONSHIP

A good dentist has been described as one who has clinical experience and skilfulness; participates in continuous professional development; is able to withstand occupational stress and financial and administrative pressures associated with general practice. Such dentists are said to be able to withstand the patients' complaints by maintaining a well-balanced distance between themselves and their patients (Kulich *et al.* 2000). However, dentists have stated that they experience both physical and psychological stress, which is associated with complaining patients, administrative problems and time pressures. They feel unable to understand their patients' difficulties and become unable to communicate freely with them. As a result the patient may experience a sense of helplessness and hopelessness. A consequence is the disruption of the treatment alliance.

If the formation and maintenance of the treatment alliance is dependent upon the dentists' and patients' communications, trust and rapport, then the factors which disrupt the treatment alliance are those which upset their ability to communicate, and to establish trust and rapport. These factors which belong to both the dentist and the patient once more run parallel with each other (fig. 2.4). They are said to include:

- **The experience and intensity of anxiety**
  For the dentist this is related to occupational stress and burnout whereas for the patient it is associated with the intensity of their dental fear and dental phobia
- **The cost**
  For the dentist it is the financial costs of providing care for the patient whereas for the patient it is not only financial costs of the treatment but also the associated costs of travel, time out of work, etc.
- **The difference between the dentists' and patients' perceptions of need**
  The differences in the meaning of need of dental treatment may cause difficulties. For the dentist perceptions of need are based upon professional training (normative need): for the patient need is related to previous dental experiences (felt need) and the ability to voice treatment wishes (expressed need) (fig. 2.4).

The dentist's understanding of factors that have the potential to inhibit the formation and maintenance of the treatment alliance is important because if difficulties arise with patients the dentist will have the ability to rectify the situation. Considering the factors related to the dentist and the factors related to the patient provides the dentist with a strategy to restore the treatment alliance and maintain the adult quality of the interaction (the real relationship) with the patient.

1.5 THE EXPERIENCE AND INTENSITY OF ANXIETY AND THE TREATMENT ALLIANCE

Occupational stress and burnout

Stress is defined as an inappropriate response to life events, an imbalance between perceived demands and ability to cope. This description suggests that almost any situation – from divorce to moving house – can trigger stress. However, more and more research has implicated the workplace and specific occupations as predisposing factors in the experience of stress. Dentistry in particular has been highlighted as a stressful occupation. Dentistry with its routine and repetitive nature was blamed, with changes in practice, litigation, aggressive and/or fearful patients, time urgency, high case loads, financial worries, problems with staff, equipment breakdowns, defective materials and poor working conditions cited as elements which increased the dentists' experience of workplace stress.

As a result, members of the dental profession reported experiencing musculoskeletal disorders, cardiovascular disease, substance abuse, depression and anxiety. However, to think that occupational stress automatically resulted in physical and psychological ill health was to ignore the role of predisposing (personality traits, environmental circumstances) and mediating (social networks) factors. These factors could influence the dentist's response to stress and moderate his/her ability to cope. Personality traits such as Type A behaviour increased an individual's vulnerability while social networks reduced the impact of stress.

When people find themselves in chronic stressful situations they become physically and emotionally exhausted and may suffer from professional burnout. Burnout has been described as:

> 'a disease of over-commitment [*associated with a*] withdrawal from work in response to excessive stress or dissatisfaction' (Cheniss 1992).

The difficulty is that it is the challenge of work, which exacerbates stress, which leads to poor work performance and ill health. The denial of occupational stress only makes things worse by increasing the likelihood of burnout. In denial the stressed individual gradually loses interest in work and job satisfaction. This leads to a further increase in stress, which in turn results in burnout. The physical and psychological signs of burnout include:

Physical signs	Psychological signs
exhaustion	touchy and irritable
gastro-intestinal problems	marked sadness
headaches	avoid commitment to care
shortness of breath	general lethargic
skin complaints	screaming/shouting
aches and pains	outbursts of anger
sleeplessness	
lingering colds etc.	

According to Gorter (2000) there are 5 types of burned out dentists:

1. The treadmill walker:

    This dentist is caught in the daily, repetitive routine of dental practice. He can see no way out and is resigned to his fate. He can see few career options and he feels that he professional development is at an end.

2. The crushed idealist:

    The crushed dentist is the disillusioned dentist. His image of dental practice has been crushed by the reality of clinical practice and can see no way forward in his career.

3. The frantic runner:

    This type of dentist tries to pack more and more into an already busy schedule. He has the tendency to become physically and emotionally exhausted.

4. The disgusted dentist:

    This dentist has come to dislike every aspect of dental practice. He realised at an early stage in his career that he had chosen the wrong profession. He finds it difficult to interact with his patients and yearns for retirement.

5. The depressed dentist:

    This type of dentist is miserable and unhappy. He finds no rest from his depressed state whether at home or at work. He neglects his family, colleagues and patients and finds little satisfaction in any aspect of his lifestyle.

Irrespective of category, the dentist who is burned out is unable to interact or communicate effectively with patients and colleagues. S/he is unable to appreciate his/her personal achievements and feels resigned to work in a profession s/he finds distasteful. His/her emotional exhaustion reduces satisfaction with work and home life, which leads to a sense of low-spiritedness.

The effects of burnout disrupt the treatment alliance as the dentist is unable to connect with his/her patients. S/he is unable to provide a caring and empathetic atmosphere and his/her lack of effective communication increases workplace stress leading to a never-ending vicious circle of stress and burnout. However, there are solutions and measures, which may be used to control occupational stress, to prevent burnout and to restore the treatment alliance.

To control occupational stress it is important to recognise and assess the demands being made upon the dentist and the dental team, to examine the appropriateness of the coping methods used and to assess the psychological and physical outcomes of the tactics used. A strategy to control occupational stress includes:

1. An assessment and evaluation of the work and environmental demands made upon the dentist and the dental team at any one time during the working day – such as work load, job performance, being responsible for patients, staff and family.

2. An assessment of the emotional outcomes of these demands – are they perceived as being threatening, irrelevant, challenging, hostile, friendly and enhancing self-esteem.

3. An assessment and evaluation of the type of controlling/coping methods used to deal with the demands – the effects of these coping strategies both in the short and long term, the outcomes and influences they have upon occupational stress, working practices and physical health. Also, behavioural methods used to diminish the effect of workplace stress are relaxation, assertiveness and problem solving.

Counselling programmes, which are tailored to the specific needs of general practitioners, have been developed to prevent burnout (Gorter 2000). The programme, which lasts for a 6-month period, allows dentists to examine issues that are associated with the exacerbation of burnout. The dentists also highlight strategies that may be used to increase assertiveness, to deal with conflict situations and to improve effective communication. Although time-consuming, the programmes have been shown to reduce emotional exhaustion and to increase self-esteem in those working in general dental practice.

Dental anxiety and dental phobia

The frightened dental patient enters the practice fearful, apprehensive and exhibiting all the physiological manifestations of anxiety. Observing the patient's behaviour and listening carefully to the patient's words the dentist will be able to decide whether this person will accept the dental treatment which is being offered and provided. The dentist's decision is made upon his/her assessment of the intensity of the patient's anxiety.

It has been postulated that a continuum exists with regard to the degree of dental anxiety which is experienced by patients attending and not attending for dental care. Swallow (1970) suggested that this continuum stretched from those patients who were relaxed to those who avoided dental care because of their fear. The majority of people were in the middle, attending despite feeling uneasy or tense. It seemed possible to suggest that as a continuum existed between relaxed to phobic reactions to dental treatment then a classification of dental anxiety with regard to dental phobia could also be made (fig. 2.5).

Dental anxiety has been defined as a fear of the unknown and is said to be situation-specific (a state anxiety). Dentally anxious patients are often able to link their present day dental fears to previous painful dental treatments. The majority of dentally anxious patients state that they are fearful of the drill, the injection and pain as a consequence of unpleasant or frightening dental experiences in childhood.

The findings from the Adult Dental Health Survey (ADHS) (Kelly *et al.* 2000) from the United Kingdom have shown that the proportion of people who stated they felt anxious about dental treatment has fallen from 56 per cent in 1988 to 49 per cent in 1998. The lower incidence in dental anxiety is said to reflect the improvement in childhood dental experiences and

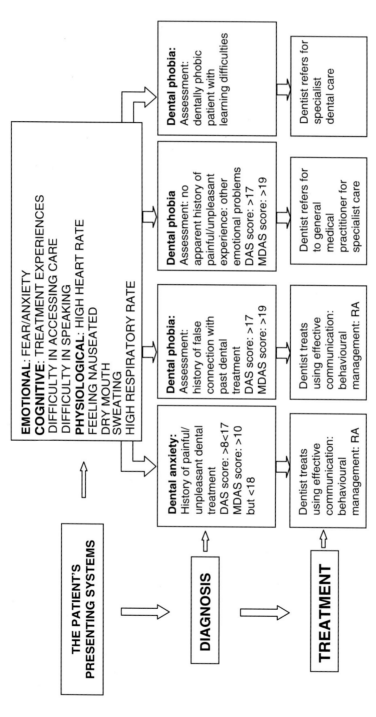

THE PATIENT'S PRESENTING SYSTEMS

EMOTIONAL: FEAR/ANXIETY
COGNITIVE: TREATMENT EXPERIENCES
DIFFICULTY IN ACCESSING CARE
DIFFICULTY IN SPEAKING
PHYSIOLOGICAL: HIGH HEART RATE
FEELING NAUSEATED
DRY MOUTH
SWEATING
HIGH RESPIRATORY RATE

DIAGNOSIS

Dental anxiety: History of painful/unpleasant dental treatment DAS score: >8<17 MDAS score: >10 but <18

Dental phobia: Assessment: history of false connection with past dental treatment DAS score: >17 MDAS score: >19

Dental phobia: Assessment: no apparent history of painful/unpleasant experience: other emotional problems DAS score: >17 MDAS score: >19

Dental phobia: Assessment: dentally phobic patient with learning difficulties

TREATMENT

Dentist treats using effective communication: behavioural management: RA

Dentist treats using effective communication: behavioural management: RA

Dentist refers for to general medical practitioner for specialist care

Dentist refers for specialist dental care

Figure 2.5 A classification of dental anxiety with regard to dental phobia.

treatment techniques. However, the proportion of people who could be classified as dentally phobic – those who stated that they would avoid dental treatment even when in pain and for whom dental anxiety was the most important barrier to accessing dental treatment – remained in the order of 10 per cent in the intervening years. Furthermore, the proportion of dental phobic people world-wide has also remained remarkably stable, again in the order of 10 per cent of the population. These epidemiological findings suggested that a differentiation should be made between those patients who are dentally anxious and those who are dental phobic. In this respect, although both dental anxiety and dental phobia presented in similar ways (that is, anxiety) it is the intensity of the affect together with identifiable, frightening, treatment experiences which permits the division to be drawn between them (fig. 2.5).

Dental anxiety

In 1946 Coriat coined the term dental anxiety. He stated that dental anxiety was a fear of the unknown, an anticipatory anxiety in which previous frightening dental experiences were relived and experienced as if they were happening in the present. Although these patients appeared crippled by their fears they were able, with help (Dailey *et al.* 2001), to accept and return for continuous dental care.

Dental phobia

A phobia is defined as irrational fear of a place or an object with avoidance of the place or object. The intensity of the anxiety is so great as to result in avoidance behaviours. No matter what anxiolytic treatments are to hand – relative analgesia, intravenous sedation or even general anaesthesia the phobic patient can refuse them all.

From in-depth work with patients it became clear that dental phobia could be considered differently to dental anxiety as dentally phobic patients made 'false connections' between experiences inside and outside the dental surgery. These experiences had elements in common. Patients who feared the local anaesthetic injection with help could link their fears to childhood experiences of painful antibiotic injections or insulin injections. The element in common was the first painful injection and the fear and pain was displaced as to all subsequent injections. This allowed a false connection to be made from injections outside to local anaesthetic injections inside the dental surgery.

A second group of phobic patients exist for whom there appears to be no obvious false connection. These patients often state that they do not remember a particularly frightening episode only that there was something that was unpleasant. Careful questioning will uncover that all is not well and that their dental phobia, rather than being a 'disease entity in its own right' is in fact a symptom of another underlying emotional difficulty. A third group of dentally phobic individuals exist. These are people who have profound learning difficulties. Their phobic reactions may or may not be a consequence of previous frightening experiences but are compounded by not understanding what is happening.

Assessment of dental anxiety or dental phobia

The assessment of dental anxiety or dental phobia is made by listening carefully to the patient's story (effective communication). Being encouraged to speak freely the patient will provide the dentist with enough information to enable the dentist to make the provisional diagnosis of dental anxiety or dental phobia.

Reliable tools for the busy general practitioner in the assessment of patient dental anxiety are a number of psychological questionnaires. These questionnaires are available for both adults and children. They are simple and easy to use and provide the dentist not only with the means of confirming his diagnosis but also as another means of engaging the patient.

The Dental Anxiety Scale (DAS)

The DAS was developed by Corah (1969) to assess adult dental anxiety. It is a four-item inventory. The questions ask about the intensity of dental anxiety when waiting for, first the day of the appointment, secondly in the waiting room, thirdly for drilling and finally for scaling. Examples of questions to assess anxiety when visiting the dentist tomorrow and waiting in the waiting room for treatment are:

- If you had to go to the dentist tomorrow, how would you feel?
  Would look forward to it as a
      reasonably enjoyable experience   ❑ [1]
  Wouldn't care one way or the other   ❑ [2]
  Would be uneasy about it   ❑ [3]
  Would be afraid   ❑ [4]
  Would be very frightened   ❑ [5]
- While you are waiting in the waiting room for your turn in the dentist's chair, how do you feel?
  Relaxed   ❑ [1]
  Uneasy   ❑ [2]
  Tense   ❑ [3]
  Anxious   ❑ [4]
  So anxious, I feel sick and
      break out in a sweat   ❑ [5]

Each question has 5 possible responses from feeling relaxed (scoring 1) to feeling anxious (scoring 5). This gives a possible range of scores from 4 to 20 with the score of 8.89 representing the population average score. Scores between 17 and 20 correspond to dental phobia.

The Modified Dental Anxiety Scale (MDAS)

The MDAS was developed in 1995 by Humphris *et al.* This is a modification of Corah's scale and includes a question about local anaesthesia. The questions assess the intensity of dental anxiety when waiting for, first the day of the appointment, secondly in the waiting room, thirdly for drilling and for scaling and finally for local anaesthesia. Examples of questions to assess dental anxiety when waiting for a dental appointment and treatment are:

- If you went to your dentist for **TREATMENT TOMORROW**, how would you feel?

Not anxious	❏ [1]
Slightly anxious	❏ [2]
Fairly anxious	❏ [3]
Very anxious	❏ [4]
Extremely anxious	❏ [5]

- If you were sitting in the **WAITING ROOM** (waiting for treatment), how would you feel?

Not anxious	❏ [1]
Slightly anxious	❏ [2]
Fairly anxious	❏ [3]
Very anxious	❏ [4]
Extremely anxious	❏ [5]

The scoring system is the same as for the DAS with total scores ranging from 5 to 25. Scores above 19 indicate dental phobia with 10.97 being the population average, for people attending general dental practitioners.

The Modified Child Dental Anxiety Scale (MCDAS)

The MCDAS was developed by Wong *et al.* in 1998 to assess children's dental anxiety when having dental general anaesthesia (DGA) or relative analgesia (RA). The questionnaire consisted of 8 items. A score of 1 relaxed/not worried to 5 very worried. The MCDAS has been modified to include faces as some children have problems with numbers (fig. 2.6). The scoring is the same as in Wong *et al.*'s (1998) original version and the scores range from 8 to 40.

Deciding on treatment

The dentist, with the patient's agreement, is now able to decide whether to treat the patient in the practice or to refer him elsewhere. This decision is dependent upon:

1. The intensity of anxiety experienced by the patient. The intensity of the anxiety may be so great that the patient is unable to accept the treatment which is being offered and provided resulting in a disruption of the treatment alliance

HOW DO YOU FEEL ABOUT:

		1	2	3	4	5
■	Going to the dentist	1	2	3	4	5
■	Having your teeth looked at	1	2	3	4	5
■	Having your teeth scraped and polished	1	2	3	4	5
■	Having an injection in the gum	1	2	3	4	5
■	Having a filling	1	2	3	4	5
■	Having a tooth out	1	2	3	4	5
■	Being put to sleep for treatment	1	2	3	4	5
■	Having a mixture of 'gas and air' to help you feel comfortable but not asleep for treatment	1	2	3	4	5

Figure 2.6 The modified child dental anxiety scale.

2. The patient's ability to understand what is being said and what is happening
3. The dentist's ability to contain the patient's fears and difficulties. The dentist may experience an increase in occupational stress again resulting in a disruption of the treatment alliance.

Some dentists, however, have the ability and enjoy treating dentally anxious patients (Dailey *et al.* 2001). These dentists use their communication and patient management skills to enable frightened patients to ventilate their fears, negotiate coping strategies and maintain the treatment alliance. According to Dailey *et al.* (2001) such dentists were characterised by:

• having time to listen to their patients
• providing accurate and clear explanations of treatment procedures and pain relief
• helping their patients cope by providing both behavioural and pharmacological management techniques (coping strategies).

The ability of the dental practitioner to use effective communication allows the treatment alliance with the anxious dental patient to be enhanced. This is reflected in the patient returning for continuous dental care; being able to speak freely of previous frightening treatment experiences and being able to cope with the intensity of his dental anxiety. Each of these actions indicate that the anxious patient has developed and maintain a positive treatment alliance with his dentist.

1.6   COSTS AND QUALITY OF CARE AND THE TREATMENT ALLIANCE

The costs and quality of dental care are inexorably linked and are further associated with perceived satisfaction of the care provided and received. Each of the factors (fig. 2.7) which contribute to the costs of care, the quality of care and perceptions of satisfaction has the ability to influence the dentist–patient relationship. For the dentist, his ability to provide high quality care for the patient, on the one hand and his ability to maintain the financial viability of the practice and job satisfaction on the other, will ultimately affect the treatment alliance. Low quality care in terms of interpersonal and clinical skills will reduce patient satisfaction causing the 'patient-consumer' to look elsewhere for care.

Dentist costs: financial and time costs

The character of general dental practice has changed. This has not only been in relation to fee and payment structures (National Health Service (NHS)

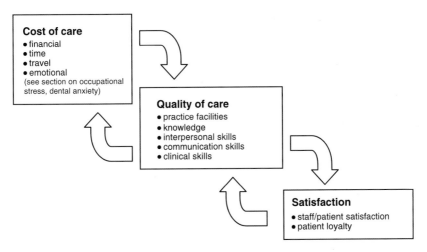

Figure 2.7 Costs, quality and satisfaction with dental care.

versus private fees) but also with the advent of 'Dental Access Centres' (salaried general practice) and 'the recent arrival of high-profile, market-driven corporate players' (Newsome 2001). These changes in general dental practice have forced practitioners to recognise the benefits of improved patient care and high quality practice (Newsome 2001).

According to Newsome (2001), in the past there has been an emphasis on 'productivity' (as in the fee per item payment structure), and this together with time urgency has been at the expense of quality patient care. Often Newsome (2001) suggests high productivity has curiously resulted in 'low fee collection', 'bad debts', 'poor cash flow' and dissatisfied patients. This has a knock-on effect as dissatisfied patients take up more practice time (increasing time urgency), demotivating the dental team reducing rather than increasing profits. Consequently high productivity can cause a financial crisis for the practices in question. The choices for dentists who find themselves in this position are not simple or easy, since there are obvious implications for their livelihoods. The degree to which financial issues are intertwined with the dental profession has been recognised in America. While the major attraction to enter the profession is financial, for many it also becomes a reason for leaving. American dentists who, despite years of training, time and effort decided to leave the profession, cited financial constraints and pressures of running a general dental practice as the main reasons.

In order to overcome financial constraints and pressures Newsome (2001) postulates a 'Service Profit Chain'. In the 'Service Profit Chain' financial success is linked to patient satisfaction, which in turn is connected to staff retention and job satisfaction. In a sense, this has a cause and effect influence upon the prosperity of the dental practice as high quality health care in general dental practice causes and consolidates improved profitability. According to Newsome (2001) for high profitability it is necessary to have high quality care as this potentiates patient loyalty, staff loyalty and staff satisfaction which in turn maintains high quality care and profitability.

Patient costs: financial costs

The financial costs of dental care have been shown to be important when considering people's ability to access dental care. The proportion of people in the UK attending for NHS dental care has fallen from 86 per cent in 1988 to 76 per cent in 1998 (Kelly *et al.* 2000). This has been associated with the gradual rise of private dental care within the UK.

The majority of people in the UK in 2003 still attend practices where NHS dentistry is provided, with over half of these adults contributing to the costs of their dental treatment. As might be expected, a cost and socio-economic status gradient existed between those who attended for private dental care compared with those who attended for NHS and those who attended for emergency treatment. Seventy per cent of dentate adults who attended the dentist on a regular basis contributed towards the costs of their dental treatment compared with 56 per cent of pain only attenders. Those who attended for private treatment contributed more than those who attended NHS practices.

Attendance at NHS practices for regular dental care was also associated with socio-economic status and geographic location. Respondents from lower socio-economic groups were more likely to attend NHS practices for the extraction of teeth compared with those from higher socio-economic groups who attended private practices for preventive care. Differences in the type of practices accessed was related to geography with 24 per cent of respondents in the south-east of England compared with 10 per cent in Northern Ireland attending private dental practices. These findings suggested that financial costs of treatment together with the socio-economic status and geography had a bearing on regular attendance and the type of care (emergency, NHS and/or private) accessed (Kelly *et al.* 2000). However despite the influence of financial costs upon accessing dental care, only 5 per cent of people (Kelly *et al.* 2000) stated that they changed their dental practice as a consequence of financial costs. These findings from the ADHS in 1998 support Newsome's (2001) views that patient loyalty outweighs the financial constraints of treatment. The dentist–patient relationships seems to be related to the satisfaction with the care the patient receives which thus promotes the treatment alliance even in the face of adversity – such as affordability of treatment costs.

Costs: travel and time costs

People's ability to access health care is associated with travelling distance. People tend to visit health care facilities within a 5 kilometre radius from their homes. This finding was reflected in the ADHS in 1998, with respondents stating that they chose a practice that was located near to their homes or work. In general majority of people travelled 3.2 kilometres to their 'family dentist'. The distance travelled was dependent upon private transport, socio-economic status and geography. People with little or no access to private transport, from lower socio-economic groups and who resided in Scotland were more likely to travel shorter distances for dental treatment.

In terms of time costs the average length of time absent from work for a dental appointment is about 2 hours (Kelly *et al.* 2000). However, the majority of respondents tended to access care outside of working hours irrespective of pattern of dental attendance, socio-economic status or geography.

Perceptions of quality and satisfaction with care

Despite people experiencing difficulties in affording and accessing dental care they remain loyal to their dentist and his/her practice (Kelly *et al.* 2000, Newsome *et al.* 2000). It seems that the key to maintaining a treatment alliance lies in the interpersonal and communication skills of the dental team. The Royal College of Surgeons (RCS 2001) in detailing the characteristics of quality care in clinical practice recognised this fact. It stated that there was a need for dental practitioners to 'put the interests of the patient first', to provide effective communication within a framework of a high knowledge base and high quality clinical care.

People who attended on a haphazard basis wished for kind, caring and communicative dental staff whereas those who attended routinely sought high quality standards of dental care. However, for those who attended on a regular basis they perceived quality of care in terms not only of high quality clinical work but also in terms of effective communication, pain control and value for money (financial costs). It seemed that the elements associated with cost and quality mediated as factors with regard to accessing, attending and accepting dental care.

Satisfaction with the care provided and received is, according to Newsome (2001), a balance between the patients' perceptions of the costs, quality of care and the dentists' ability to deliver. Newsome (2001) maintains that the discussion of the fees is a critical juncture in providing quality dental care. The fee or financial costs must be openly discussed in order to prevent dissatisfaction on the part of the patient (fears of exploitation) and the dentist (fears that his work is undervalued). If the discussion of the fee is not tactfully negotiated then patients may decide to leave the practice and go elsewhere.

Interpersonal skills and the ability of the dentist to encourage discussion about fees and associated concerns will, according to Newsome (2001), enable patients to accept the dental treatment that the dentist is offering and providing despite concerns with regard to affordability. However, in order to achieve and maintain the treatment alliance with the patient the dentist must provide high quality care in terms of interpersonal and communication skills, knowledge base and high quality clinical skills.

1.7 PERCEPTIONS OF NEED

Dental health care needs are sensitive to many psycho-social influences such as socio-economic status, previous experiences, level of education obtained, knowledge, attitudes, fears, expectations, satisfaction and so forth. Consequently, dental health goals will be different for individuals within the same population, for people from different geographic locations and different ethnic groups. Considering that patients and dentists may differ in one, some or all of these psycho-social/cultural influences, it is of little surprise that misperceptions exist between lay and professional perceptions of dental health care needs. Therefore, although the dentist can clinically define the patient's treatment needs this might not reflect the patients' true wants, needs or wishes. The dentist may have one perception while the patient has another. Problems occur for the treatment alliance when these two perceptions of need are at odds with one another. The degree to which the dentist and patient agreed or disagreed, in this regard, has been shown to influence the treatment alliance. The requirement for health professionals, in general and dentists, in particular, to be aware of the potential for a mismatch allowed Bradshaw (1972) to postulate a 'Taxonomy of Need' to understand the concept of health care need. Bradshaw (1972) proposed 4 different types of need:

(i) Normative need
The professionally defined need. This need is identified by dentists, when they clinically diagnose disease or perceive a fall in acceptable standards of personal health care. Normative need is dictated by the dentist's professional training. Difficulties arise when this is based on value judgements which may reduce the patient's satisfaction with the care received.

(ii) Felt need
This is what patients feel about their health needs. This is the lay perception of health needs, it is what the patient wishes, wants and what he feels should be done. This is often different to professionally defined need and may bring the dentist into conflict with the patient.

(iii) Expressed need
These are the needs that patients communicate to the dentist both in words and deeds. These are different from felt needs which the patient may feel but be unable to tell the dentist about. Dentists must be able to encourage and give the patient the opportunity to express their felt needs. Barriers to communication may be related to dental anxiety or fears of the dentist's criticisms.

(iv) Comparative need
The last category of need is 'comparative need'. This concept of need relates more to the management of the practice rather than the interpersonal relationship with the patient. Nevertheless an appreciation of comparative need (the identification of the characteristics of the population using the practice service compared with the characteristics of those with similar characteristics who do not) may provide the dentist with a means of increasing accessibility for the population which is served by his practice.

It would seem reasonable to propose that the treatment alliance will be enhanced or inhibited in accordance with the extent to which the patient's and dentist's perceptions of need are matched or mismatched. The patient will either be satisfied or dissatisfied and this will affect the stability of the treatment alliance. However, Ong (1993) voiced caution with this simplistic view of professional–lay mismatch. She has suggested that since health care needs are part of an individual's lifestyle it means that they may be traded off against other more urgent or important felt needs. This may be illustrated by patients whose business engagements or family matters take precedent over attending for dental appointments. At other times these same patients will make arrangements and go to extraordinary lengths to attend. The idea that mismatch perceptions are somehow fixed in time ignores the dynamic nature of the treatment alliance. An awareness of this provides the dentist with an insight and a technique to stabilise and strengthen the treatment alliance. This may be achieved by using appropriate and effective communication skills to encourage the patient to ventilate their treatment wishes and to enter into discussions with regard to treatment planning. Dentists who follow this style of patient management are able to divert and/or to modify ideal treatment plans to respond to the specific needs of the individual patient.

1.8 ASSESSMENT OF PROFESSIONAL AND LAY PERCEPTIONS OF NEED

The realisation that differences exist between lay and professional perceptions of need has paved the way for a number of oral health indices to evolve. These are different to the usual indices used in clinical practice such as the 'Plaque Index' or DMFT. The newer indices acknowledge that a relationship existed between psychological, social and physical health (Freeman 2000). Furthermore they attempted to assess how an individual's psychological and social functioning could be restricted and limited by the impact of oral disease. The Oral Health Impact Profile (OHIP) (Locker *et al.* 2001) was the first to assess how psychological (feeling self-conscious) and social (avoidance of social situations) functioning was affected by the impact of physical oral disease. From this earlier work shortened versions of OHIP (14 items compared with the original 49 items) evolved together with other instruments which assessed the impact of dental disease upon social functioning. Many of these indices have been used in dental health surveys (Kelly *et al.* 2000) but have not been applied to the general practice setting. A requirement remained, for a professional–lay need index to be available for general practice which could promote communication, include the patient in his/her oral health care and strengthen the treatment alliance.

The Oral Health Index and Oral Health Score

The 'Oral Health Index' (OHX) (Burke and Wilson 1995), a short index suitable for the time constraints associated with general practice, is ideal for this purpose. The OHX is an 8-item instrument which assesses oral health. The first three items assess felt and expressed needs – the patients' experience of pain; their ability to chew; the appearance of their dentition. The remaining 5 items assess the normative need – the oral mucosa; the occlusion; caries status; 'wear and tear'; periodontal health. Each item is scored individually to produce an overall score which is the percentage of the maximum achievable. Scores may range from 0 (poor oral health) to 100 excellent oral health. The OHX has been adapted by a UK-based private dental capitation company, Denplan (Winchester, UK), to form the Oral Health Score (OHS) (fig. 2.8).

FELT/EXPRESSED NEED ITEMS	QUESTIONS ASKED	SCORING	OUTCOME
1. PAIN	Experiencing pain ?	No pain = 8 Minor pain = 4 Disruptive pain = 0	⬆
2. CHEWING ABILITY	Chew an unrestricted diet?	Unrestricted diet = 8 Minor problem = 4 Major problems = 0	Improved communication + strengthening of treatment
3. APPEARANCE	Concerns about appearance?	No concerns = 8 Minor concerns = 4 Major concerns = 0	alliance ⬇
NORMATIVE NEED ITEMS	**PROFESSIONAL CRITERIA**	**SCORING**	**OUTCOME**
1. ORAL MUCOSA		No lesions detected = 8 Lesion needing observation = 4 Lesion requiring treatment = 0	If score =0 then refer for specialist care
2. OCCLUSION	10 teeth present in each jaw: (natural or artificial teeth)	10 teeth present in each jaw and oppose each other = 8 Otherwise score = 0	⬆
3. CARIES STATUS	Mouth divided in sextants:	Any sextant free of active decay = 4 Any sextant with tooth with active decay requiring restoration = 0	Improved communication + strengthening of treatment
4. TOOTH WEAR	Mouth divided in sextants:	Any sextant free of tooth wear = 2 Any sextant with tooth with active decay requiring restoration = 0	alliance
5. PERIODONTAL HEALTH	Mouth divided in sextants:	Start with score of 24. From this score delete the Basic Periodontal Examination score for each sextant	⬇

Figure 2.8 Oral Health Score.

Community Index of Denture Treatment Need

Fiske *et al.* (1998) highlighted the importance of emotional factors and the expressed needs of the denture wearer with regard to treatment outcome. They (Fiske *et al.* 1998) showed that patients, after many years, experienced an unhappiness associated with the loss of the natural dentition. The degree of this distress was correlated with their ability to wear dentures and to inter-act easily with acquaintances, friends and family (Fiske *et al.* 1998). It was clear that dentists needed to appreciate the extent to which emotional factors and social health impinged on the lives of complete denture wearers. The necessity to be able to assess the expressed (treatment wishes) and felt (emotional and social) needs of complete dentures patients was recognised (McNaugher *et al.* 2001a,b) and this gave rise to the development of a community index of denture treatment need (CIDTN).

The CIDTN assesses both normative and felt/expressed need for and experi-enced by complete denture wearers (McNaugher *et al.* 2001a,b). The index was designed for use in the dental surgery or domiciliary setting. The value of the index was that it assessed both professional and lay aspects of denture treatment need providing the dentist with an indication of the need to replace dentures.

The index is in two parts. The first part is the normative need assessment based upon questions, for example, the state of repair; centric jaw relation-ship; articulation and occlusal balance of the dentures (McNaugher *et al.* 2001a). (Table 2.2).

Table 2.2

State of repair	Upper	Lower
Satisfactory	☐[0]	☐[0]
Fractured acrylic	☐[1]	☐[1]
Tooth lost	☐[1]	☐[1]
Has been repaired	☐[1]	☐[1]
Other	(please state)	
Centric jaw relationship		
Satisfactory		☐[0]
Unsatisfactory/unbalanced		☐[1]
Articulation and occlusal balance		
Acceptable		☐[0]
Unacceptable		☐[1]

The second part is an assessment of the patients' felt and expressed need. Questions in this part of the index included:

[1] psychological health
[i] Generally speaking do you feel anxious or frightened?
YES   ❏ [1]   NO   ❏ [0]
[ii] Generally speaking do you feel miserable or depressed?
YES   ❏ [1]   NO   ❏ [0]
[iii] When you feel anxious and/or depressed can you still do house work/jobs around the house?
YES   ❏ [1]   NO   ❏ [0]
[iv] When you feel anxious and/or depressed do routine tasks (like housework) take more effort?
YES   ❏ [1]   NO   ❏ [0]

[2] social health
[i] Do you like how you look when you are wearing your dentures?
YES   ❏ [1]   NO   ❏ [0]
[ii] Generally speaking how satisfied are you with how your dentures look?
Very satisfied   ❏ [1]
Fairly satisfied   ❏ [2]
Can't say   ❏ [3]
Fairly unsatisfied   ❏ [4]
Very unsatisfied   ❏ [5]
[iii] Do you meet with friends and/or family?
YES❏ [1]   NO❏ [0]

If **yes**: how often to you meet with friends and/or family?
Each day   ❏ [1]
Twice weekly   ❏ [2]
Weekly   ❏ [3]
Monthly   ❏ [4]
Less often   ❏ [5]

[3] perceptions of oral health
[i] Generally speaking how satisfied are you with your dentures?
Very satisfied   ❏ [1]
Fairly satisfied   ❏ [2]
Can't say   ❏ [3]
Fairly unsatisfied   ❏ [4]
Quite unsatisfied   ❏ [5]
[ii] Do you experience pain when wearing your dentures?
YES   ❏ [1]   NO   ❏ [0]
[iii] Do you experience pain when eating with your dentures?
YES   ❏ [1]   NO   ❏ [0]
[iv] Does your mouth feel dry?
YES   ❏ [1]   NO   ❏ [0]
[v] Do you have painful ulcers in your mouth?
YES   ❏ [1]   NO   ❏ [0]
[vi] Do you experience any problem when speaking with your dentures?
YES   ❏ [1]   NO   ❏ [0]
[vii] Do your dentures feel loose?
YES   ❏ [1]   NO   ❏ [0]

Research has shown that the CIDTN is a valid means of assessing the treatment needs of patients who wear complete dentures (McNaugher *et al.* 2001*b*). Patients who reported satisfaction with their dentures perceived their oral health as good, interacted easily with family and friends and had no discernible treatment requirements. As the inclusion of patient's treatment wishes and needs has been shown to be a prognostic factor in positive treatment outcomes it is advisable to encourage patients to participate in the decision-making process and include assessments of expressed and felt need when treatment planning for complete denture wearers.

Effective communication, whether using the spoken word or with the help of questionnaires, assists the dentist in the assessment of felt and expressed need and is an essential part of the treatment planning process. The ventilation of potential treatment-related problems allows the treatment alliance to be strengthened at the expense of factors that would disrupt its formation. The dentist's awareness of the patient's wishes and needs together with normative treatment need provides the means by which the dentist and patient can cooperate more together towards a common goal. The recognition of potential treatment-related problems allows an open discussion and provides a pathway by which the patient may be encouraged to participate in the decision-making process. The negotiated treatment plan formed with the approval of both participants sustains the treatment alliance. Working in this dynamic way allows the dentist to discover the patient's treatment wishes, fears and concerns and results in the maintenance of the treatment alliance.

1.9   CONCLUSION

In conclusion, the aim of this chapter was to demonstrate the importance of the dentist–patient relationship and specifically the 'treatment alliance' in the management of the patient. Factors which affect both the patient and the dentist have been used by way of illustration to show how social and psychological factors sway the treatment alliance. The ability to balance these psychosocial factors which strengthen and sustain the treatment alliance, on the one hand, against those that have the potential to disrupt and destroy the treatment alliance on the other, relies upon the dentist's communication and management skills. The ability to communicate effectively, to recognise potential pitfalls and to be aware of the disruptive elements (e.g. occupational stress), which may inhibit the formation of the treatment alliance, can assist in strengthening the interaction between dentist and patient. The need to develop, maintain and sustain the treatment alliance may be considered as the touchstone of primary dental care as it provides a pathway by which the dentist and patient can work together towards the common goal of oral health.

REFERENCES

Bradshaw J. (1972) Taxonomy of need. In (ed. G. McLachlan) *Problems and Progress in Medical Care*. Oxford: Oxford University Press.

Burke FJT, Wilson NHF. Measuring oral health: an historical view and details of a contemporary oral health index (OHX). *International Dental Journal* 1995;45:385–370.

Cherniss C. Long-term consequences of burnout: an exploratory study. *Journal of Organisational Behaviour* 1992;13:1–11.

Corah NL. Development of a dental anxiety scale. *Journal of Dental Research* 1969;48: 596.

Coriat IH. Dental anxiety: fear of going to the dentist. *Psychoanal Rev* 1946;33:365–7.

Dailey Y-M, Crawford AN, Humphris GM, Lennon MA. Factors affecting dental attendance following treatment for dental anxiety in primary dental care. *Primary Dental Care* 2001;8:51–6.

Falkum E, Førde R. Paternalism, patient autonomy, and moral deliberation in the physician-patient relationship. Attitudes among Norwegian physicians. *Soc Sci Med* 2001;52:239–48.

Fiske J, Davis DM, Frances C, Gelibier S. The emotional effects of tooth loss in edentulous people. *British Dental Journal* 1998;184:90–3.

Freeman R. (2000) *The Psychology of Dental Patient Care*. London: BDJ Books.

Goold SD, Lipkin M. (1999) The doctor-patient relationship: challenges, opportunities and strategies. *Journal of General Internal Medicine*;

Gorter RC. (2000) Burnout among dentists: identification and prevention. University of Amsterdam: Thela Thesis.

Greenson RR. (1967). *Technique and practice of psychoanalysis*. London Hogarth Press. 1985.

Humphris GM, Morrison T, Lindsay SJ. The modified dental anxiety scale: validation and United Kingdom norms. *Community Dental Health* 1995;12:143–50.

Kelly M, Steele J, Nuttall N, Bradnock G, Morris J, Nunn J, Pine C, Pitts N, Treasure E, White D. (2000) *Adult dental health survey. Oral health in the United Kingdom 1998*. London: HMSO.

Kulich KR, Berggren U, Hallberg LR-M. Model of the dentist-patient consultation in a clinic specialising in the treatment of dental phobic patients: a qualitative study. *Acta Odontol Scand* 2000;58:68–71.

Locker D, Matear D, Stephens M, Lawrence H, Payne B. Comparison of the GOHAI and OHIP-14 as measures of the oral health-related quality of life of the elderly. *Community Dent Oral Epidemiol* 2001;29:373–81.

Massé R, Légaré F. The limitations of a negotiation model for perimenopausal women. *Sociology of Health and Illness* 2001;23:44–64.

McNaugher GA, Benington IC, Freeman R. Developing a schedule of normative denture treatment need. *Gerodontology* 2001a;18:41–50.

McNaugher GA, Benington IC, Freeman R. Assessing expressed need and satisfaction in complete denture wearers. *Gerodontology* 2001b;18:51–7.

Newsome PRH. (2001) *The Patient-centred Practice: a Practical Guide to Customer Care*. London: BDJ Books.

Newsome PRH, Wright GH. Qualitative techniques to investigate how patients evaluate dentists: a pilot study. *Community Dentistry and Oral Epidemiology* 2000;28:257–66.

Ong BN. (1997) *The Practice of Health Services Research*. London: Chapman-Hall.

Senate of Dental Specialities (2001) *Good Practice in the Dental Specialities*. London: Royal College of Surgeons.

Swallow JN. Fear and the dentist. *New Society* 1970;5:819–21.

Szsaz TS, Hollander MH. A contribution to the philosophy of medicine. *Arch Int Med* 1956;97:582–92.

Wong HM, Humphris GM, Lee GT. Preliminary validation and reliability of the Modified Child Dental Anxiety Scale. *Psychol Rep* 1998;83:1179–86.

3 Practice building – relationships within the practice

1.0 THE DENTAL TEAM

The term 'dental team' has become synonymous with primary dental care. What at one time seemed a vague term has gained greater clarity in recent years. According to Whateley (1998) it describes how a group of dental health professionals come together to work towards a common goal providing dental health care for their patients:

> '[*The dental team is*] made up of a group of individuals able, willing and prepared to work with others while taking responsibility for their contribution to the dental care of individual patients'.

1.1 PROFESSIONALS COMPLIMENTARY TO DENTISTRY

Nurses and receptionists

The image of the *dental team* has, therefore, changed. The term no longer represents the single-handed dentist working with a dental nurse but rather the dentist as team leader, working in a multi-handed practice in unison with a practice manager, receptionists, dental nurses, hygienists and so forth. Reflecting this change, the General Dental Council in 1998 revisited the Report of the Inquiry into Education and Training of Personnel Auxiliary to Dentistry ('The Nuffield Report' 1993) to provide clear and concise guidelines on the training and clinical duties of professions complimentary to dentistry (PsCD).

In their 1998 report the General Dental Council emphasised the importance of PsCD:

> 'All groups of PCD should be trained, qualified and statutorily registered with the General Dental Council' ... with 'The needs of the patient and the protection of the public [*being*] of paramount importance'.

In the past the dental team may often have comprised a dentist and a nurse who also acted as receptionist. This was achievable because the dentist may have worked standing up, with the patient sitting upright. Much of the treatment may have been prosthetics rather than operative. Today, treatment may be much more demanding and varied, with the patient lying supine for treatment and the concomitant need for a chairside assistant. A nurse is therefore a vital member of the team, centrally involved in the care of the patient and the dispensing and mixing of the wide variety of dental materials which form the dentist's armamentarium.

Given the nurse's involvement at the chairside, a receptionist will also be required. A basic knowledge of the procedures carried out in the surgery is essential for this team member: indeed, a training as a dental nurse may be useful in order to facilitate appropriate scheduling of appointments, although the time allotted for each patient should be the clinician's responsibility.

The ratio of receptionists per dentist in a practice depends on practice busyness. However, it is generally accepted that one trained and competent receptionist can manage the appointment scheduling, telephone answering etc. of two dentists.

Other PsCD

Today, the dental team will often include PsCD. This recently introduced term comprises dental nurses, hygienists, therapists, orthodontic therapists, dental technicians and clinical dental technicians. These are the members of the modern dental team. It therefore becomes apparent that today and tomorrow's dentist will be the leader of a substantial team, with each member having different capabilities and responsibilities.

There appears to be a growing shortage of dentists in the UK. The challenge is to determine the effect of a number of factors on this shortage. These include:

- the scale of early retirements by dentists, and retirements due to ill health
- the extent of part-time practice, in particular by the increasing number of female dentists
- to gauge whether technology will improve the efficiency of the average practice,
- whether the move towards privately funded dentistry will increase,
- whether the demand for elective and aesthetic procedures will continue to rise (Barry 2001), and
- whether water fluoridation will become more widespread, and if so, the effect of this.

These are many imponderables, but, notwithstanding the last, the trend in the UK would appear to be towards increasing practice busyness.

The demand for treatment could, of course, be coped with in a number of ways:

- by increasing the number of dental students, but this would take time to organise, and would be difficult to reverse if demand decreased, since universities would have had to increase the number of teaching staff
- by importing dentists from abroad
- expanding the duties of hygienists, and/or increasing the numbers of therapists, and/or expanding the duties of qualified dental nurses.

By giving increased responsibilities to the latter groups their job satisfaction will be improved and these PsCD will look on their jobs as long-term careers rather than as a short-term option, which seems to be the case for some dental nurses today.

From history, it is only at a time of reduced demand that dentists become resentful of the 'competition' that PsCD provide – a situation seen in the US in the early 1970s (Meskin 1977). That is not the case today. By delegating some procedures to PsCD, dentists who choose to do so should be able to concentrate on more complex forms of treatment.

A further advantage which follows an increased role for PsCD could be a reduction in the cost of providing simple treatment, as incomes of PsCD are less than dentists. Since the average working life of an auxiliary is less than that of a dentist, increased flexibility could be also built into the system. There is a paucity of data on the attitudes of dentists to PsCD, but results of a 1993 survey indicated that 20% of dentists would oppose the employment of therapists in practice (Hay and Batchelor 1993), while in 1982, 27% stated that they would oppose such a move (Woodgrove and Harris 1982). Since younger dentists were found to be more supportive of the concept of delegation to auxiliaries, it could be argued that support for PsCD will grow (Hay and Batchelor 1993). In countries where therapists work in practice, such as Canada, Australia and New Zealand, the experience seems satisfactory, while in many states of the US, expanded duty nurses have worked successfully for many years. In the UK, the General Dental Council has authorised the introduction of therapists into dental practice. It therefore seems only a matter of time before the dentist is seen as the leader of the team of dental nurses, hygienists, therapists, orthodontic therapists, dental technicians and clinical dental technicians, prescribing treatments for patients and delegating those that are appropriate to the appropriate members of the team. This concept will require a difference in attitude and skill from the dentist of the past who was used to carrying out most of a patient's treatment, to being a manager of the patient's care, in turn managing the team members who are providing it. Management training may therefore become a requirement of the undergraduate dental curriculum.

The dentist–laboratory relationship

The advice of Mr Colin Lee for this section in acknowledged
For indirect restorations and prostheses, the general dental practitioner requires the assistance of a dental technician. This is a partnership in which each has specific responsibilities. The clinician must produce a preparation which is adequate in terms of resistance and retention form, and take a satisfactory impression, but also allow the technician sufficient space to build the restoration, notwithstanding the need to provide the technician with all the information needed to fabricate the restoration or prosthesis. Dental technicians tend to specialise in prosthetics or restorative treatments and some general dental practitioners will work exclusively with the same technicians for many years. The general dental practitioner may base his/her choice of technician on a number of factors. These may include the technician's qualifications and ability to produce the required restoration or denture, cost,

and location/convenience. However, the relationship is ultimately based on a mutual trust built through the provision of patient treatment together. Prior to the patient's attendance for a preparation appointment, it is often helpful for the clinician and technician to have discussed the case: this is obviously made easier if they are located conveniently to each other. Prior to treatment, the technician and clinician should discuss, with the aid of articulated, surveyed (where appropriate) study casts, and/or a diagnostic wax-up:

- the interabutment space,
- ridge dimensions and contour,
- potential interocclusal space in centric relation and excursive movements,
- pontic shape,
- bridge design,
- crown or bridge material,
- partial denture design

It is the dentist's responsibility to provide the technician with all the information required to produce the restoration or prosthesis. This is helped by the use of a well-designed laboratory form, with boxes or spaces for all essential information. In addition to the factors listed above, the following information should also be provided:

- Patient information – name, age and sex
- Method of funding of restoration
- Shade(s), with shade map where required
- Shade of underlying tooth (of special relevance to veneer and dentine-bonded crown cases)
- Stage to be returned
- Date of fit, or next stage, appointment
- Type of teeth, size, mould, for dentures

Any additional patient requests should also be communicated to the technician. Pre-operative photographs may be of value, both in denture cases and crowns and bridges. In this respect, recently introduced shade matching equipment uses digital photography. Other recently developed shade matching devices are colourimeters or spectrophotometers: such equipment should minimise the possibility of a shade mismatch, although a correct shade match is dependent on (i) the correct choice of shade by the dentist, and (ii) the correct shade build up in the laboratory.

In conclusion, the development and maintenance of a good relationship between dentist and technician is central to the achievement of excellence in crown work and fixed and removable prosthodontics. Additionally, as the technician will be aware of the incidence of remakes or early failures associated with the techniques and materials that s/he is using, because dentists will communicate these to the laboratory, our technicians are usually in possession of early knowledge of the potential for success of a given technique. Communication between dentist and technician helps ensure that such knowledge is extended to patient care.

1.2 THE DENTAL TEAM WORKING TOGETHER

The dental team therefore can now be thought of as a sum of its members and not as a group of individual players. Considering the dental team in this way allows an appreciation that the people working together in the practice provide it with its unique character and practice philosophy.

However, achieving this unified approach requires the dentist as team leader to have a variety of management skills that reflect the diversity of her position within the practice. These include the following:

- the establishment of effective communication skills,
- the ability to respond positively to team members,
- the provision of a platform for planning and identifying practice target goals, and
- the motivation of team members to work together towards the formulated plan.

The dentist by producing formulated plans can identify specific goals for each team member as well as ensuring the quality of the dental health care provided in the practice. Doing so affords the dentist an opportunity to give positive and appropriate feed-back to each team member as a means of team development. In this way the staff are encouraged to develop and evolve their skills both in the clinical arena and in their inter-personal dealings with others. The dental team now changes and with the recognition of the need for practice quality assurance becomes an effective and efficient working structure. The process of team development has been described as empowerment with the developed team being characterised by:

> 'a high degree of interdependence, self-determination, competence, commitment and ... concern about the quality of work being performed'

> (Wilson 1998)

1.3 WHAT MAKES A QUALITY DENTAL TEAM?

Quality assurance is a means of ensuring that the minimum standards of quality in dental health care are achieved. A quality dental practice is a reflection of the quality of the members of its dental team. At the highest level, quality is determined by Government policy with the need for training to be legislated and recognised and for team members to be registered with statutory bodies such as the General Dental Council. Quality assurance at the practice level includes structure, process and outcomes as descriptors of minimal acceptable standards of practice work and patient care. This is the next level of quality assurance – the *structure* of the practice, practice routines (*process*) and how the practice and its personnel are perceived by patients (*outcomes*) (Table 3.1) (Burt *et al.* 1999).

Although Burt *et al.* (1999) describe quality assurance as structures, processes and outcomes this is an artificial divide as each aspect of quality is inter-linked. The structure of the practice (such as the surgery equipment) will affect job satisfaction both at the chair-side and in the reception. At the chair-side effective equipment **(structure)** will improve the efficiency of clinical routines **(processes)** while recognition **(management)** of the nurse's skills will increase job satisfaction and patient care **(outcomes)**. In the reception up-to-date computer hard and software will affect the efficiency of processes within the practice. These include practice protocols (administration), patient records (process), appointments and recall protocols (outcomes). The ability of

Table 3.1 Quality Assurance in the General Practice Setting (Burt *et al.* 1999)

STRUCTURES OF THE PRACTICE	PROCESSES WITHIN THE PRACTICE	PRACTICE OUT-COMES
Facilities	*Management*	*Patient satisfaction*
1. setting	1. practice	*Oral health status*
2. physical layout	2. personnel	1. oral hygiene
3. access	3. patient	2. tooth loss
		3. periodontal health
Equipment	*Records*	4. caries experience
1. surgery	1. content	5. prevention
2. instruments	2. completeness	
3. dental materials	3. availability	*Completion of treatment*
4. autoclaves	4. legibility	1. time
		2. appropriate
Personnel	*Diagnosis*	
1. training	1. appropriate	*Recall pattern*
2. interpersonal skills	2. documentation	1. method of recalling
3. job satisfaction	3. thoroughness	2. frequency
4. in-service training		3. needs at recall
	Treatment planning	
Administration	1. written	
1. formulated plans	2. sequencing	
2. practice protocols	3. appropriate	
3. appraisal systems		
	Treatment	
	1. appropriate	
	2. timeliness	

the dentist to develop practice protocols, working strategies and to provide quality working conditions has been shown to influence employee continuity within general practice.

Considering quality assurance as an integral part of the functioning of the dental team, provides the dentist with a framework to plan, develop, evolve and maintain the practice. Formulated plans as part of the administrative structure of the practice allows regular appraisal of the quality of practice work. The appraisal or staff assessment provides a third level of quality assurance. Using team members' job specifications as the basic requirement of practice work allows the dentist to appraise the staff's clinical and interpersonal skills, while negotiating their future professional goals. By using such strategies the dental team can evolve into a coherent working group.

1.4 STRATEGIES OR ACHIEVING QUALITY IN THE DENTAL TEAM

The dentist, as team leader or facilitator, must be able to provide a working environment which allows the development of the quality of the dental team. The expertise needed to perform this task is associated with socia and group skills. Group skills operate at interpersonal (social) and collective (group) levels. They require the dentist to be able to communicate effectively, to plan regular practice meetings and to have constructive staff appraisals in order to motivate and enable staff to achieve their personal professional goals. However the skills associated with groups are different to those associated with individuals on a one to one basis. In order to understand how people interact within the group setting it is important to consider how people form groups, operate within a group structure and what happens when people leave the group. A useful way of thinking about group dynamics is to use Tuckman's Stages of Group Life (Whateley, 1998). The Stages of Group Life describes how groups go through a variety of different stages from the moment people meet for the first time until they meet together for the last time. It is suggested that a group goes through five stages. The five stages (fig. 3.1) are getting started (*forming*), settling in (*storming*), getting down to work (*norming* and *performing*) and moving on (*mourning*).

Effective communication within the dental team uses the same verbal and non-verbal format as those described for working with patients. The types of questioning, the ability to explain and listen carefully are all needed when communicating effectively with staff members. However, the aim of the interaction is different as it is continually changing not only on a daily basis but also as new staff members are chosen and become integrated into the dental team. Therefore the skills and emphasis in communication

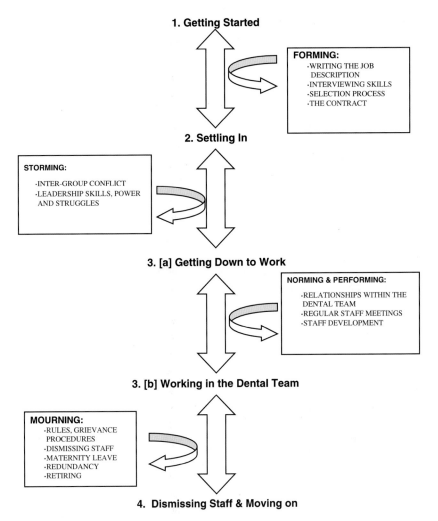

1. Getting Started

FORMING:
- WRITING THE JOB DESCRIPTION
- INTERVIEWING SKILLS
- SELECTION PROCESS
- THE CONTRACT

2. Settling In

STORMING:
- INTER-GROUP CONFLICT
- LEADERSHIP SKILLS, POWER AND STRUGGLES

3. [a] Getting Down to Work

NORMING & PERFORMING:
- RELATIONSHIPS WITHIN THE DENTAL TEAM
- REGULAR STAFF MEETINGS
- STAFF DEVELOPMENT

3. [b] Working in the Dental Team

MOURNING:
- RULES, GRIEVANCE PROCEDURES
- DISMISSING STAFF
- MATERNITY LEAVE
- REDUNDANCY
- RETIRING

4. Dismissing Staff & Moving on

Figure 3.1 Strategies for achieving quality in general dental practice.

change accordingly. Acknowledging the dynamics of the group provides the dentist with strategies to use as a facilitator, to promote quality within the practice (Table 3.1). The need to be proficient at complying job specifications may be essential when forming the group or looking for new members of staff but less useful when in the norming and performing stages. The ability of the dentist to adapt her communication skills needed to promote quality may be different to those needed when interacting with patients. The adaptation of Tuckman's schema for working in the general practice setting explains the need for dentists as facilitators and team leaders to remain flexible when planning and developing strategies to achieve the quality dental team.

1.5   GETTING STARTED

Writing the job description

The first communication the dentist has with new staff is written in the form of the advertisement and job description. The job specification will define the necessary training, qualification and requirements needed for the position (Blair 1997). Looms (2000) suggests drawing up a job specification based on what is essential and what is desirable in the potential employee (for example a dental receptionist) (Table 3.2). In addition the dentist must consider the requirement for this new position and how the new staff member will fit in with the practice philosophy and style.

Once the essential and desirable characteristics have been recognised the specific duties to be undertaken by the new member of staff must be identified. In describing a job specification for a dental hygienist, Blair (1997) clearly sets out all duties which must be undertaken. He describes general duties which include:

> 'providing clinical care of patients as requested by the dentist, within the framework outlined below [clinical duties, education and motivation and practice management].'

In addition Blair (1997) itemises what must be included in each aspect of the work – in the preparation of the surgery for operation (for example, ensuring sterilisation of equipment and disinfection of services, setting up trays), the general care of patients (for example, all dental care is prescribed by the dentist, good manners, clarification of position within the dental team), clinical duties (for example, examination of periodontal tissues, screen, observe and record changes in oral health status, pit and fissure sealants), dental health education (OHI, motivation) and practice management (accurate clinical records, effective communication with other members of the team, continuing professional education).

Table 3.2   Essential and desirable characteristics for the potential employee (Looms 2000)

Characteristics	Essential characteristics	Desirable characteristics
Experience in practice	Minimum 6 months	1–2 years A-levels
Qualifications	GCSEs	Spreadsheets 1–2 years
IT ability	Word processing	Teamwork experience
General office experience	Interpersonal skills	
Group skills		
Appearance	Smart at all times	

Interviewing skills

From a clear and precise job description the short-listing or selection for interview is made easier. The division of the job specification into essential and desirable characteristics allows the dentist to choose potential practice employees from a number of applicants. Once this part of the selection process has been completed the dentist must decide upon the interview format. This period of time between the end of the short-listing period and the interview itself allows the dentist to design the interview (James 1999), to write to referees, to request that the short-listed candidates bring copies of their qualification certificates, to decide who will be on the interviewing panel and to check upon the legitimacy of the interview format and potential questions with regard to employment legislation.

Although the interview process is a two-way process it is characterised by a power differential between the employer and potential employee. In order to reduce this inequity, James (1999) has suggested that a simple form should be designed containing all the questions which should be asked to each candidate in turn with at least two people on the appointments panel (Looms 2000). It has been recommended that the questions should be divided into professional (for example: 'What do you want in the future?' or 'Would you take this job if it was offered to you?') and personal factors (for example: 'What would you do if a patient complained about the care they had received?'). The division of questions into previous working experiences, attitudes towards working with patients provides the basis for assessing whether this person has the potential to become an integral member of the dental team.

During the interview Looms (2000) advises the use of a three-step process first based upon the use of closed, then open and finally focused questions. Looms (2000) suggests that this unusual sequence of asking questions allows candidates to relax, gain confidence and give their best at interview.

The closing part of the interview is important as it demonstrates to the candidate that the employer perceives the work situation as a two-way process. It is in the final stages of the interview that candidates are invited and provided with the opportunity to ask questions of the interview panel. This allows them to raise issues important to them (for example: in-service training) and to clarify aspects of the job (for example: salary).

The selection process

After the interview all the information about the potential employees has been gathered and the dentist together with the other members of the selection panel will be able to make a decision. Looms (2000) stresses how important

THE THREE-STEP PROCESS

In the following example the dental nurse's knowledge and skills when working with anxious patients is being assessed:

Dentist: 'Have you worked with anxious patients before?' (CLOSED QUESTION)

Candidate: 'Yes'

Dentist: 'What types of treatment do you know of to reduce dental fear?' (OPEN QUESTION)

Candidate: 'Patient management, RA'.

Dentist: What do you mean by patient management?' (FOCUSSED QUESTION)

Candidate: Talking to the patient, finding out why they are frightened, telling them what's going on. It's important to have everything ready for the dentist, that reduces the patient's time in the chair. I think that helps to reduce their fear too. They know they can manage OK. I am there to help the dentist and the patient.

the job specification is in the selection process. In addition, using this strategy for staff selection provides the basis for staff development and appraisal. It is from the job specification that a definition of a threshold of competency has been made and which allows the candidates to be compared. There are several consequences of this process; first, one candidate may obviously be the best; secondly, more than one candidate fulfils the job specification and levels of competency required and thirdly, none of the candidates reach the threshold required in the job specification. In the first scenario the best candidate will be offered the position. In the second case a decision must be made with regard to which of the potential employees will complement the practice philosophy. In the last situation no one should be employed and the position re-advertised.

Contract of employment

Within 2 months of being appointed a contract must be given to the new employee. A contract is a written statement of the terms and conditions of employment. This must contain names of the employer and employee, the date of commencement of employment and about its continuity, job title and description of duties, place of work, scale/rate of remuneration, incremental intervals, hours of work, holiday and holiday payments, maternity leave, sickness and sick pay, pension and position under the Social Security Pensions Act 1975, length of time of notice, grievance procedure, disciplinary rules and procedure and details of agreements which affect the terms and conditions of employment.

1.6 SETTLING IN

Intergroup conflict

The new staff member should be provided with a contract and practice policy documents. The contract must comply with employment legislation. Practice policies must include discipline, grievance procedures, equal opportunities, disability, sickness and confidentiality. It has been recommended that new members of the dental team are given a trial period of 3 months. This again reflects the two-way process of the work situation. The dentist as employer can assess the new individual's work and how they are settling in, and the new member of staff can assess how they feel about working in the practice. In this respect the practice and the new employee are both keeping their options open.

From the point of view of the new person and the dental team they join, time is needed to settle in. The settling-in period is important as it takes time for the new person to be at ease with the new work environment, different clinical routines and for the staff to welcome and include her in the group. In terms of group dynamics, the new person is orientating herself to the work situation and while appearing hesitant may seem to be dependent upon the dentist or practice manager. It is during this time that the other staff members may withdraw and appear to be envious or jealous of the incomer.

The settling-in period is also associated with increases in emotionality which may be manifested as occupational stress. Occupational stress is characteristic of this phase as unrealistic expectations together with role conflict and ambiguity are additional burdens placed upon the dental team. Role ambiguity is associated with a change in employment status within the practice. This may occur when a dental nurse becomes employed as a practice manager in the same practice. Conflict, associated not only with the demands of the new position but also how they are perceived by their peers, may lead to disagreements, hostility and anxiety. The stressful situation is exacerbated when poor communication exists between staff as this results in rumour, leading to unaired grievances and mistrust. The settling-in process may truly be stormy.

Leadership skills, power, and struggle

The dentist's group leadership skills come into play during the settling-in period. The dentist must be able to view the difficulties encountered by staff with empathy and objectivity, remaining (above all) impartial. The dentist, as team leader, is at the centre of the practice communication network and by communicating effectively with the staff can allow grievances to be aired, ways forward to be discussed and negotiated. The quality of the relationships between staff members will be enhanced by effective management and good communication during this phase.

Argyle (1981) calls the skills the dentist must use when faced with such situations as 'handling skills'. He states that 'handling skills' are in fact a special type of social skill in which the dentist as leader must be aware of the dynamic quality of the relationship with the staff. Argyle (1981) suggests that the dentist's relationship with the staff lies on a continuum which stretches from cooperation to assertion, with each type of intervention necessary for the smooth running of the dental practice. Assertive interventions must be within the confines of the professional interaction and it is essential that these are made in a polite and non-patronising manner. The dentist as task leader has to maintain this position while keeping on friendly terms with the dental team.

Within the cooperation–assertive continuum there are four main types of intervention. These are altering the meaning of the demands felt and being made by the dental team, solving the problems, regulating occupational stress and collective coping. Bailey (1985) proposes that communication is pivotal. The most important communication skill when identifying and altering the dental team's demands is to listen to the concerns, worries and fears of those involved. Once the demands have been identified and their perceived meaning located within the wider structure of the practice it becomes possible for the problem to be solved. Inherent within the problem-solving intervention is the recognition of the team members' strengths and weaknesses. The need to acknowledge difficulties encountered in accepting a new member of staff, changes in clinical regimes and the wish to acquire appropriate professional skills regulates occupational stress and assists in the development of informal collective coping strategies.

In the storming period the dentist must be able to withstand the attacks made upon her as leader and use her handling and social skills to reduce inappropriate reactions, regulate work-place stress and increase self-esteem in her employees. Working in this way provides the basis for group cohesiveness and solidarity and paves the way for collective coping which is characteristic of the norming stage of group development.

1.7 GETTING DOWN TO WORK AND WORKING IN THE DENTAL TEAM

Relationships within the dental team

The relationships within the dental team have now entered a calmer period in which informal and formal social networks within the practice have been formed. Collective coping uses the social networks formed during the storming phase which are themselves a reflection of the group's new found cohesiveness. The group now starts to work as a team, with each player providing a part of the whole. However, interactions between members of the dental team do not remain static but are dynamic, constantly changing, responding to needs in the internal environment of the dental practice and the external environment of the society.

The effect of the internal surgery environment upon perceptions of job satisfaction of dental nurses is well known. The relationship with the dentist is in a constant state of flux. Research findings suggest that the dental nurse who feels her clinical work is appreciated has greater job satisfaction and less work-place or occupational stress. However when dentists make increasing and inappropriate demands, dental nurses admit to feeling like 'dental housewives' (Gibson *et al.* 1999) with the demands ('paying dental suppliers' or 'cleaning the surgery') being made upon them similar to those experienced in their home lives. Similarly dental hygienists have stated that the dentist's recognition and appreciation of their clinical skills increases job satisfaction, reduces their occupational stress and is linked to their remaining in the same practice for many years.

Changes in the number of women qualifying in dentistry and entering general practice may have an effect upon relationships within the dental team. Research (Gjerberg and Kjølsrød 2001) examining the interactions between women health professionals has demonstrated that they are different compared to those between male doctors and female nurses. According to Gjerberg and Kjølsrød (2001) women doctors in an attempt to obtain clinical assistance and avoid conflict make 'friendly relationships with the nurses'. This leads to problems and entanglements when the women divulge personal details and/or emotional difficulties. Equivalent situations may exist for women dentists and dental nurses (Freeman *et al.* 2004). An awareness of these difficulties and problems may help in maintaining the cohesiveness of the dental team in the norming phase which may be shattered by disagreements between staff members.

The interpersonal relationships in this stage of group development are tenuous and easily affected by adversity from factors beyond and within practice. Stresses from the world external to the practice may disturb relationships at work resulting in a return to the storming phase. The dentist's leadership skills must be used to reduce tensions and work-place stress. In some instances the role of the dentist is to listen and support individuals who are experiencing difficult times in their personal lives. In describing how best to deal with a bereaved member of staff, Toombs (1989) suggests that the dentist must listen to the individual and provide support as necessary. The remaining staff are in a better position to provide personal support and express their concerns for the bereaved individual. This proposed split in group function allows the dentist as team leader to provide a secure base from which staff members can accommodate and monitor the feelings and behaviour of their colleague.

Sexual harassment

In recent years concerns about the appropriateness of relationships between staff members of the dental team have been raised specifically in relation to sexual harassment in the work-place. Sexual harassment is any sexual or sex-based behaviour which is unwelcomed by staff. It includes overt sexual actions, conditioning pay and/or promotion in exchange for sexual favours and sexual comments or remarks that result in an uncomfortable or stressful atmosphere in the practice (Weinstein 1994, Capen 1997). Research has suggested that sexual harassment is 'a significant problem for women in the [*dental*] workforce to-day' with over half of female hygienists interviewed reporting that they have experienced harassment from their male dentist-employers (Garvin and Sledge 1992).

Problems arise as many of those being harassed may feel unable to voice their unease or communicate their embarrassment. In view of this Chiodo *et al.* (1999) have described the dentist's ethical and legal obligations towards the employees. They stated clearly that the individuals in the dental team are protected by law against this inappropriate behaviour and as such the legal implications of either participating or allowing it to persist in the dental practice are great. The need to protect staff from sexual harassment is paramount with the responsibility lying with the dentist as employer. The trust and confidence felt by the staff is dashed to be replaced by mistrust and suspicion. The dentist must be proactive and establish practice policy and provide appropriate protocols to prevent and manage sexual harassment. It is imperative that the dentist uses handling and social skills to provide an atmosphere in which formal and informal networks can be re-established. One way this can be achieved is by organising regular meetings.

Regular staff meetings

Staff meetings allow the cohesiveness of the dental team to be consolidated during the norming and performing phases of the group interaction. It does this by providing an opportunity for the dentist to praise staff members and acknowledge their achievements in a public forum. This setting allows people individually or collectively to air grievances and concerns about practice developments. Practice meetings are therefore important as they provide a platform from which the concerns and anxieties of individual staff members may be raised and in which the views of the dental team as a whole may be voiced.

Meetings should be held at regular intervals in which practice developments such as the delegations of administrative and/or clinical tasks can be discussed. The ability of the dentist to delegate responsibilities to the employees is associated with leadership style. The skills involved are related to an open rather than a hierarchical style of management. Open styles of management are associated with regular practice meetings. Although raised by the dentist the delegation of responsibilities is a team decision. In this way the cohesiveness of the group is perpetuated by formal networking which promotes motivation and personal development of the dental team.

The more that the dentist can listen and explain the reasons for change the more likely the staff will be to respond in a positive and constructive manner. The dental team will gradually become motivated perceiving their position in the practice as something essential and worthwhile. Scott (2000) has suggested that listening to the views of staff assists them in negotiating their work priorities when asked to take on extra duties. The use of a check-list of questions may help in assessing whether the dental team is being adequately motivated. The questions include (Scott 2000):
'Do you communicate or plan as a team how to work together?'
'Do you socialise together as a team?',
'Does anyone thank you for your work in the surgery?'
'How do your working conditions compare to the norms?', and
'Is there mutual support within the team?'.

The dentist supports the team by listening to concerns, focusing on the positive and so improving productivity and reducing work-place stress. Working in this way reduces the likelihood of de-motivation during the performing phase by increasing work motivation.

Practice meetings may also take the form of staff appraisals with the individual's job description being used as the minimum level of quality. It is from this benchmark specification that the appraisal of administrative and/or clinical work is made. The first appraisal of staff should occur within nine months of starting the new position. The individual will have completed a phase of consolidation in which she will have an understanding of the work involved and her place within the dental team. She will now be able to identify the strengths and weaknesses and the need for further professional training (Horner 1995).

The dentist must provide guidance and direction during the appraisal process and this may be achieved by listening carefully to the individuals' aims for personal growth within the constraints of their home-work interface. The four-item strategy '**GROW**' (Lansberg 1996) is ideal as a means of appraisal in such situations. It allows the dentist and staff member to identify professional **G**oals, the **R**eality of alternative **O**ptions and time-related objectives with regard to staff development to be scheduled (**W**rap-up).

The time spent during the appraisal procedure allows staff members to raise personal issues which may affect their work and which they would not wish to raise in a more public arena. These may include concerns about salary, worries about working hours and personal difficulties experienced at home. The dentist, once cognisant of these facts, can re-enter the goal setting strategy and re-negotiate time-related work objectives with the individual.

Using the appropriate questioning and explaining skills the dentist can place the desired professional goals within the realm of the practice philosophy with alternative options being raised as necessary in order to plan and implement staff development.

Staff development

With the end of the appraisal and/or staff meeting the planning stage closes and with a course of action having been tabled. It is during this time that the dentist has demonstrated commitment to staff development and continuing education for all in order to maintain the quality of the dental team and uniqueness of the practice. Staff development is a method of continuous education within an employment setting. Its focus is to update and/or increase knowledge and skills to improve performance which complements the practice policies and developments (Horner 1995).

Horner's (1995) model of staff development relies upon the appraisal process as a means of assessing the needs of the dental health professional (fig. 3.2). This is a special form of planning and assessment cycle in which the beneficiaries are the patients attending for continuous dental care. Needs assessment during the appraisal process allows staff members to identify aspects of their work which could be enhanced by continuous education. The planning and development phases interconnect by producing an implementation formula which takes into account factors which will enable (e.g. practice support and/or resources) and/or inhibit (e.g. practice policy, home constraints) the outcome of the educational programme. The desired outcomes for the dental practice may include: increase in knowledge (e.g. smoking cessation programmes in dental practice); skills (e.g. interpersonal skills) and attitude (e.g. acceptance of a new practice policy). Consequently the practice, the staff and patients benefit as the 'competencies' and 'performance' of dental team members improve.

Any changes that may be planned in practice policy mean that in-service training is doubly necessary, not only to maintain the quality of dental health care but also because continuous education of the dental team has become mandatory. Dentists intending, for instance, to provide sedation services for their patients must employ dental nurses who have the Certificate in Dental Sedation Nursing. Therefore at staff appraisal meetings dental nurses willing to undertake a course of study may be identified and a negotiated plan of action formulated and implemented. The desired outcome is the Certificate in Dental Sedation Nursing, an increase in the dental nurse's specialist knowledge and skills, increased clinical performance and competencies which advance and improve not only self-esteem and professional standing but also the dental health care of the practice's patients (fig. 3.2).

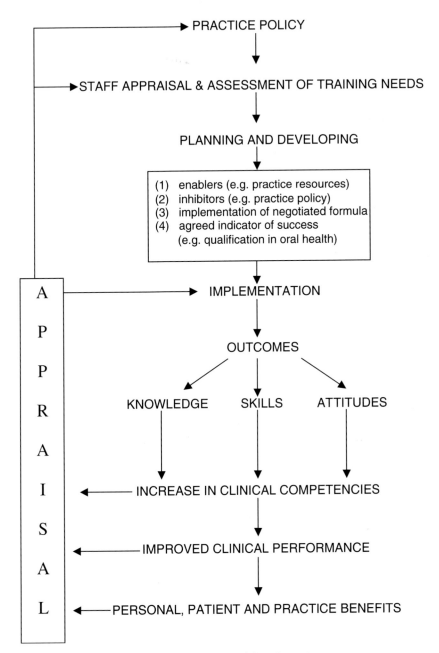

Figure 3.2 Model of staff development for general dental practice.

The final part of the staff development is an assessment or appraisal of the entire process. This is not an arduous task as each part of the process may be assessed individually, with questions directed to assess the implementation of the action plan, the level of clinical competency and the benefits accrued to the individual, the practice and patients. In addition this model of staff development provides an appraisal framework which is responsive and flexible to changes in practice personnel, philosophy and policy.

The dental practice is now, in terms of group dynamics a mature and empowered working group. It may be characterised by the philosophy of the dental practice, the quality of its dental care, the strong emphasis on its proactive and open management style and the trust and reliance each member of the team has upon one another. The vitality of the dental practice is kept alive by the enthusiasm of its practice principal who acknowledges the strengths of the dental team while improving the quality of care by staff development.

1.8 DISMISSING STAFF AND MOVING ON

The final phase of group dynamics is the mourning stage. This phase is associated with feelings of loss and bereavement as people prepare to leave the practice. People leave for a number of reasons which include finding a new position in another practice, maternity leave, redundancy, retiring or being dismissed.

For the individual the mourning stage is associated with unhappiness at leaving and excitement at moving on to a new position. As the person works out the period of notice he may be less committed to the practice and the remaining staff may minimise their colleague's achievements so reducing their sense of loss. However in some instances the individual who is leaving has been dismissed and this may cause a variety of feelings in the staff ranging from guilt to relief. The need for the dentist as employer to respond appropriately to this situation will allow the group to use their collective coping strategies to reduce their feelings at this time.

Dealing with disciplinary matters and grievance procedures

The concerns about discipline may come from the dental team or from the staff member. This is an important distinction as the dentist as employer must act differently in accordance with the source of the grievance. Needless to state, communication skills are central to dealing with complaints from or about staff members. However unlike previous interactions with the dental team the dentist is constrained by legal rules and guidelines governing grievance, disciplinary and dismissal procedures. It is essential, therefore, that the dentist has complied with these regulations and given the employee a contract together with a set of employment rules.

Staff members may feel that they have been poorly treated and it is hoped that the matter can be dealt with by the dentist in the usual way. However, when this proves impossible the employee may resort to the grievance procedure. This is a two-stage procedure in which the member of staff has the opportunity to have the problem resolved as quickly and effectively as possible. The entire proceedings should last no longer than three days resulting in an amicable solution for all concerned.

The rules of employment contained within the contract must be written in a clear and concise manner. The rules should include items such as 'timekeeping, providing reasons for absence, accurate completion of time sheet, protection of practice and patient's property, smoking, serious offences (e.g. breach of confidentiality, theft, violence), immunisation etc. The rules will provide a baseline from which evidence about a complaint associated with disciplinary matters may be founded. It is not the role of this section to deal in depth with the intricacies of disciplinary matters but to state that the alleged offences must be investigated thoroughly, that the employee must be notified of the complaint in writing and that the legal guidelines must rigidly be adhered to as all employees working for one year in a practice have full employee rights. Employees are legally entitled to being accompanied at the disciplinary interview by a trade union representative and/or colleague. Furthermore the dentist as employer must ensure that the individual is given an explanation of any penalty imposed and given the opportunity to appeal.

The dentist must attempt to pre-empt difficulties which may result in dismissal. Occasionally (e.g. gross misconduct) this is impossible, but in other circumstances (e.g. poor work performance) the dentist may attempt to counsel the staff member. Sometimes despite the dentist's best efforts the staff member fails to improve and at this point a verbal warning will be given. The dentist as employer is bound by employment legislation and must give two further warnings in writing. The reasons and the burden of proof for fair dismissal (e.g. bad time-keeping, rudeness, carelessness, conduct, poor performance etc.) lies with the dentist. This is a trying experience for all concerned and the dentist's ability to support the staff through this period is a reflection of leadership skills.

Maternity leave, redundancy and retiring

Women members of the dental team in the UK are entitled to 18 weeks statutory maternity leave and 40 weeks additional maternity leave. The expectant mother must give 21 days notice of her maternity leave, two weeks of which must be before childbirth. Although this is a different set of circumstances compared with dismissal it may have the same outcome with regard to the mourning phase. The staff member may lose interest in work and look forward to the baby's birth.

Redundancy of staff occurs when the dentist has decided to reduce his workforce. This may be a result of change of practice philosophy, the practice closing and/or the dentist retiring. For whatever reason it is necessary for the dentist as employer to hold a special practice meeting in order to consult with the dental team. The dentist must state the reasons for the redundancies, provide written criteria for selection (e.g. skills, qualifications, standards of performance, time-keeping) and inform the staff that meetings will be arranged to discuss the matter with interested parties. Working in this way allows staff members to make their own decisions with regard to the redundancy package and gives them the opportunity to plan for new professional developments.

Members of the dental team may leave when they have decided to retire. This may be the end of an era for a practice with the decision having been made to sell the practice to another dentist. The excitement of retiring may be mingled with feelings of sadness at the loss of colleagues and staff. For the staff there may be a romanticising about earlier times and concerns about how the practice will change and alter.

The mourning period is a time of sadness and change which heralds the start of a new group cycle. With the new member of staff new group dynamics evolve and the dental team returns once more into the forming phase of group development.

2.0 HEALTH AND WELFARE OF THE DENTIST AND HIS/HER TEAM

There is a commonly held view that dentistry is a stressful profession, based on statistics collected in the 1970s (Howard et al. 1976). It has been postulated that dentists, and, by inference, their staff, face a unique set of problems such as time-related pressures, fearful patients, financial worries and staff problems (Cooper et al. 1987). Additionally, dentists may experience potential occupational hazards related to the materials used in the surgery along with other potential risks such as aerosols and particulate debris. More recently, data published in 1999 from the Government Actuary on the National Health Service Pension Scheme (1989–1994) have indicated that the frequency of premature retirement due to ill health is 4 times as prevalent among dentists at age 42 years as in medical doctors (who might be considered an equivalent group in terms of qualifications and training).

Data presented by Burke and co-workers (1997) have identified reasons for premature retirement of dental practitioners on health grounds, with musculoskeletal disorders and stress-related illnesses being the most consequential groups of diseases (Burke et al. 1997). Other workers have found that dentists had significantly lower mental well-being than a comparable group from the general population (Cooper et al. 1987). Conversely, results of a US study published in 1976 have indicated that dentists' mortality rates were lower than other professional groups for the most common causes of death, with 73% of deaths occurring after the age of 64 (Orna and Mumma 1976). Nevertheless, the results of an evaluation of UK general dental practitioner stress levels indicated that one in three of the respondents were considerably dissatisfied with their job (Cooper *et al.* 1987). Negative patient perceptions and scheduling problems were noted as the primary stresses relating to poor job satisfaction. Additionally, sources of stress experienced by general dental practitioners have been identified by Blinkhorn (1992) as being the payment system, a feeling of being undervalued and the feeling of being trapped in a practice until retirement (Blinkhorn 1992). Scully and co-workers (1990) compared standardised mortality ratios (SMR) among dentists and demonstrated that dentists have lower SMRs than the general population in the UK and USA, with 73% of dentists living beyond the age of retirement. It would therefore appear that dentists are not, in general, at increased risk from illnesses, but, nevertheless, a proportion of these physical and mental illnesses result in premature retirement. It is therefore essential that dental healthcare professionals take steps to ensure that they are not affected by occupational illnesses. No data are available in respect of occupational illnesses affecting dental nurses, hygienists or auxiliaries, but it could be assumed that, as they work in a similar environment as the dentist, they could be similarly affected.

Musculoskeletal problems

Physical stress may be caused by body distortions due to incorrect working posture, poor vision of the operating area, and difficult access to the operative site (Paul 1991). Musculoskeletal problems accounted for 30% of diseases which caused premature retirement of dentists, with cervical spondylosis, arthritis/spondylitis of the spine and arthritis of the hands being the most common causes of premature retirement in this group (Burke *et al.* 1997). Learning and maintaining correct posture while operating on patients is therefore essential to the avoidance of musculoskeletal problems, since musculoskeletal pain and disability may be caused by distortions which may produce tensions in joints and their attendant muscles.

Common faults in sitting posture of dentists include (Paul 1991):
1. dental chair is too low or too high
2. dentist works too far away from the chair
3. chair back and head rest are not horizontal, so dentist must lean forward, causing overflexion of the spine
4. excessive twisting of the dentist's cervical and thoracic vertebrae, caused by dentist attempting to view facial surfaces of posterior teeth by direct vision.

A basic rule is to have the patient horizontal, with his/her mouth at or around the same height as the clinician's elbow, when the clinician's upper arm is relaxed. Ideally, the dental healthcare professional should not have to twist, bend or distort in order to treat the patient.

The ideal working posture for restorative and periodontal procedures has been described by Ellis Paul in 1991 as the 'finger-control posture' (figs. 3.3 and 3.4), which is similar to that used for any type of precision work outwith dentistry. The criteria for this are:

1. the long axis of the torso should be vertical
2. the line of the shoulders should be horizontal
3. the hip line should be horizontal
4. the thighs should be splayed outwards at no more than 30° to the mid-sagittal plane
5. the upper arms should hang vertically and the elbows be in contact with the side of the rib-cage
6. the forearms should be elevated, pivoting at the elbow joint
7. the fingertips should be at the focal distance of the operator's eyes
8. the head should be tilted forward by no more than 30° to the vertical

Other operative procedures, such as those involved in removable prosthodontics, may be readily accomplished with the patient sitting upright and the dentist standing in a good upright posture without distortion. There should be nothing inherently stressful about the standing posture apart from the physical fatigue if it is adopted for a long period of time (Paul 1991). With regard to seated height, the lower border of the thigh should be parallel to the ground, thereby maintaining the correct concavity of the lumbar curve and reducing pressure on the abdominal cavity (Paul 1991) (fig. 3.4).

Members of the dental team increasingly spend time in front of a computer screen, accessing, for example, data relating to patients, information on products and techniques as well as finding 'evidence' in respect of success rates of techniques and materials. It is therefore important that

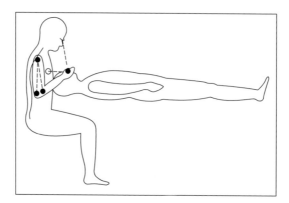

Figure 3.3 Criteria for finger-control posture (after Paul E, 1991).

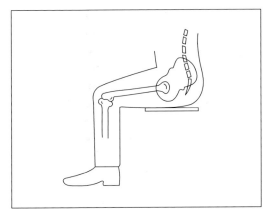

Figure 3.4 Sitting with the upper border of the thighs at 15° to the horizontal produces a correct femur-trunk angle of 105° and the correct lumbar curve is preserved (after Paul E, 1991).

those using computers also maintain appropriate posture in front of the screen (fig. 3.5).

Avoiding stress

The difficulties dentists experience with occupational stress have been examined in Chapter 2, Section 1.5 with regard to the treatment, alliance and the dentist–patient relationship. However, to reiterate, stress-related problems have been related to a lack of an efficient working system, time

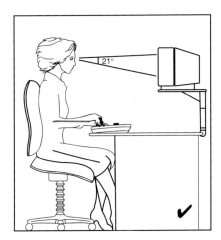
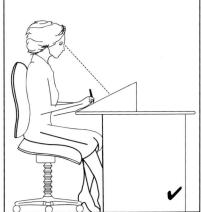

Figure 3.5 Healthy sitting to avoid back pain.

pressures (incorrect use of the appointment book), delays in the work sequence and breaks in concentration and pressures on time, fearful patients, financial worries and staff problems. Avoidance of stress therefore could be achieved by avoiding these difficulties, whenever possible. Regarding time pressures, ideally, spaces should be left for patients who phone for urgent or emergency appointments and the time left for each clinical operation should be realistic rather than optimistic. Avoidance of financial worries might be achieved by a dentist assessing the level of earning that he hopes to make, to decide the number of hours he wishes to work per annum, examine the practice overheads and then calculate and set an hourly rate by which patients are charged. Stress may be avoided by using materials and laboratories which perform predictably and by employing and developing staff who are responsible and trustworthy and with good attendance records. In this respect, consideration could be given to a practice bonus scheme, whereby staff with no absences in a given time are rewarded. In the twenty-first century, stress is probably endemic among all in the UK who are working. However, sensible working patterns, employment of good staff and looking after their personal development, having a realistic financial strategy and using predictable materials and laboratories can all contribute to the smooth working of a dentist's day list and keep stress at a manageable level.

Allergies to dental materials

Resin-based materials, in particular, have the potential to sensitise members of the dental team who come in contact with them. Glove wearing does not necessarily help, as some frequently used resins may penetrate latex gloves in less than 10 minutes. Good resin hygiene is therefore paramount, with the dental nurse and dentist striving to ensure that bonding agents do not contaminate gloves. Recently developed materials, with unidose presentations, may be advantageous in this respect. It could be considered advisable that resin-bonding agents are not be allowed to touch the patient's gingival tissues or mucosa in order to reduce the risk of the patient developing an allergy to one or more of the resin constituents, although there is little evidence that this could occur. It is worth adding that dentists, on postgraduate hands-on courses or at exhibitions, should not handle resin-based materials with their bare hands for risk of sensitisation.

Allergy to natural rubber latex affects between 5% and 10% of healthcare workers, a considerably higher figure than for the general population (Hill *et al.*, 1998). Fortunately, for the dental healthcare worker who has developed such an allergy, satisfactory alternatives, in the shape of nitrile gloves, are now available. A smaller proportion of patients may be allergic to natural rubber latex, in particular, healthcare workers, and those with congenital urinary tract deformities. These patients should be treated at the earliest appointment of the morning so that the risk of latex particles in the surgery atmosphere is minimised, using natural rubber latex-free gloves and rubber dam.

Mercury hazards

Mercury toxicity may manifest itself as kidney disease, eventually leading to kidney failure, tremor and memory loss. There is recent evidence that dentists have a higher incidence of kidney disease and poorer short-term memory than a control group, although this was not correlated to the level of mercury vapour in the dentists' surgeries. Nevertheless, almost half of the surgeries tested had mercury vapour levels greater than the UK Occupational Control Standard (Ritchie *et al.* 2002).

These data point to the need for stringent control of mercury in the dental surgery.

Boredom

It has previously been considered that one of the problems faced by the practising dentist is the potentially routine and boring nature of the job (Cooper *et al.* 1987). There is no question that the placement of amalgam restoration after amalgam restoration may present little in the way of mental and philosophical stimulation, even if every different patient presents with different problems of management. It is therefore beholden to the clinician to maintain an interest in postgraduate education, learning about new techniques, and expanding the range of clinical skills that he/she possesses–'pushing back the comfort zone'. Many successful established practitioners will develop specialised clinical interests, which may not be at the level of specialist on a General Dental Council list, but which may provide additional mental stimulation. Research, writing, training a vocational dental practitioner or lecturing are among other additional interests which may help prevent boredom.

3.0 CONCLUSION

In conclusion, the aim of this chapter was to provide strategies to develop and maintain the quality and health of the dental team in general dental practice. It is proposed that the dentist is the key individual who determines the quality of the dental health care provided for the patients. Effective communication skills and a knowledge of group dynamics allows the dentist as team leader to set the ground rules of quality for the practice. Doing so enables the dentist and the team to evolve into a coherent, inter-dependent, competent and motivated group concerned with the quality of care they provide for their patients.

REFERENCES

Argyle M. (1981) *Social Skills and Health*. London: Methuen.

Bailey RD. (1985) *Coping with Stress in Caring*. Oxford: Blackwell.

Barry VJ. Solving the shortage. *J Am Dent Assoc* 2001;132:728–9.

Blair DJ. Writing a job description or contract for a dental hygienist in dental practice. *J NZ Soc Periodontol* 1997;82:40–5.

Blinkhorn AS. Stress and the Dental Team: a qualitative investigation of the causes of stress in general dental practice. *Dent Update* 1992;19:385–87.

Burke FJT, Main JR, Freeman R. The practice of dentistry: an assessment of reasons for premature retirement. *Br Dent J* 1997;182:250–4.

Burt BA, Eklund SA, Ismail AI, Ekland SA, Fletcher J. (1999) *Dentistry, Dental Practice, and the Community*. Philadelphia: W.B. Saunders. Corp.

Capen K. Harassment issues should be dealt with before they become problems. *Can Med Assoc J* 1997;156:1577–9.

Chiodo GT, Tolle SW, Critchlow C. Sexual boundaries in dental practice: part 2. *General Dentistry* 1999;47:552–227.

Cooper CL, Watts J, Kelly M. Job satisfaction, mental health and job stressors among general dental practitioners in the UK. *Br Dent J* 1987;162:77–81.

Freeman R, Gorter R, Braam A. Dentists interacting and working with Woman Dental Nurses: A Qualitative Investigation of Gender differences in Primary Dental Care. *British Dental Journal* 2004;196:161–165.

Garvin C, Sledge SH. Sexual harassment within the dental office in Washington State. *J Dent Hyg* 1992;66:178–84.

General Dental Council (1998) *Report of the Inquiry into Education and Training of Personnel Auxiliary to Dentistry*. London: HMSO.

Gibson BJ, Ekins R, Freeman R. The Role of the Dental Nurse in General Practice. *British Dental Journal* 1999;186:213–15.

Gjerberg E, Kjolsrod L. The doctor-nurse relationship: how easy is it to be a female doctor co-operating with a female nurse? *Soc Sci Med* 2001;52:189–202.

Government's Actuary Department. Report by the Government Actuary on the National Health Service Pension Scheme 1989–1994. London, 1999, The Stationery Office.

Hay IS, Batchelor PA. The future role of dental therapists in the UK: a survey of District Dental Officers and general practitioners in England and Wales. *Br Dent J* 1993; 175:61–6.

Hill JG, Grimwood RE, Hermesch CB, Marks JG. Prevalence of occupationally related hand dermatitis in dental workers. *J Am Dent Assoc* 1998;129:212–16.

Horner B. (1995) *Handbook of Staff Development. A Practical Guide for Health Professionals*. Melbourne: Churchill-Livingstone.

Howard JH, Cunningham DA, Rechnitzer P, Goode RC. Stress in the job and career of dentists. *J Am Dent Assoc* 1976;93:630–6.

James KR. Ask the experts: how can I find the right employees? *J Am Dent Assoc* 1999;130:1101–3.

Landsberg M. (1996) *The TAO of Coaching*. London: Harper Collins.

Looms S. Recruit in haste, repent in leisure. *Dental Business* 2000;4:14–17.

Meskin LH. Too many dentists? If so, what then? *J Dent Educ* 1977;41:601–5.

Orner G, Mumma RD. Mortality study of dentists: final report, prepared for the National Institute for Occupational Safety and Health. Philadelphia, Temple University Health Sciences Center, School of Dentistry, 1976.

Osborne D, Croucher R. Levels of burnout in general dental practitioners in the south-east of England. *Br Dent J* 1994;177:372–7.

Paul JE. Team Dentistry 1991. Martin Dunitz, London.

Ritchie KA, Gilmour WH, MacDonald EB, Burke FJT, McGowan DA, Dale IM, *et al. Occup Environ Med* 2002;59:287–93.

Scott S. (2000) Team organisation. *Independent Dentistry*. September: 37–9.

Scully C, Cawson RA, Griffiths M. *Occupational Hazards to Dental Staff*. London, British Dental Association, 1990.

Toombs ME. The dentist and the bereaved co-worker. *J Can Dent Assoc* 1989;55:457–8.

Whateley B. (1998) *A Very Special Team: a Practical Guide to Developing and Motivating a Dental Team*. London: BDJ Books.

Weinstein BD. Sexual harassment: identifying it in dentistry. *J Am Dent Assoc* 1994;125:1016–21.

Wilson CK. Team behaviours: working effectively in teams. *Semin Nurse Manag* 1998;6:188–194.

Woolgrove J, Harris R. Attitudes of dentists towards delegation. *Br Dent J* 1982; 152:335–40.

4 Practice building: the need for excellence in treatment

Many aspects of dental practice contribute to overall patient satisfaction. This may include comfortable surroundings and helpful, efficient staff, but these will count for nought if the treatment which is provided is not of a good standard. Excellence in treatment therefore is central. This may be considered to include correct diagnosis and treatment planning, health promotion, prevention rather than intervention, and, where intervention is indicated, the use of minimally invasive (MI) treatment techniques. It also includes the efficient diagnosis and treatment of dental emergencies, knowing when and whom to refer, and the ability of the clinician to manage the increasing number of patients with special needs. This chapter includes sections on treatment planning, oral health promotion and prevention, MI techniques, dental emergencies, the management of patients with special needs, the evidence-based concept for treatment and clinical governance.

1.0 TREATMENT PLANNING (N H F WILSON, A J M PLASSCHAERT AND F J T BURKE)

Many factors may influence priorities in the provision of adult dental care. Among these are:
- changes in society,
- changes in oral health,
- the patient's dental expectations,
- life expectancy gains and the retention of increasing numbers of teeth throughout life, and,
- changing views on the desirability and benefits of good oral health.

As a result, the impressions gained by clinicians from the initial patient interview and the clinical examination have assumed new importance. Effective treatment planning demands a thorough knowledge and appreciation of a patient's history and oral health status, based on objective rather than subjective data pertaining to the condition, function and comfort of all elements of the stomatognathic complex, in the context of whole body health. Effective treatment planning must be based on an holistic view of the patient, an understanding of patients' expectations and aspirations and an appreciation of their felt and expressed needs. For a successful outcome, it is therefore essential from the outset that the dentist 'gets to know' the patient (See Chapter 2). Subsequently, appropriate examinations, tests and investigations must be completed in a systematic approach to provide detailed knowledge of the status, function and comfort of the dentition. The reliability and objectivity of these tests and examinations may be improved by auditing the outcome of examinations and clinical testing. Furthermore, it is essential that the clinician is aware of the potential for success of any given procedure, and is aware of the factors influencing its success, i.e. that the clinician is able to adopt an 'evidence-based' approach to the planning of patient treatment.

1.1 THE PATTERN OF ATTENDANCE

The order of treatment may differ between operators and patients, with the status of the patient (re-attender or new) and the patient's pattern of attendance being important determinants. Moreover, the treatments prescribed and their order of provision may depend upon the perceived likelihood of the patient becoming or continuing to be a regular attender.

The irregular attender

The irregular attender may be more likely to present with an acute problem requiring immediate treatment, although regular attendance does not preclude presentation as an emergency. In either case, emergency treatment needs should not be dealt with without consideration of definitive care, as a decision regarding the treatment of the emergency may influence the treatment options in subsequent care.

The regular attender

The frequency of regular attendance, sufficient to maintain oral health, may vary according to the patient's disease incidence and previous treatment need. It may be considered that the regular attender is a patient:

'who can be relied on to return for continuing care without undue encouragement in the absence of signs or symptoms of active disease'.

By contrast, the irregular attender may be considered a patient:

'who attends only when s/he perceives a need for treatment'.

The frequency of attendance for the regularly attending patient is dependent on the patient's dental history and susceptibility to dental disease. For example, the patient with low levels of active disease, good oral hygiene maintenance, limited physiological wear and healthy mucosa should not require dental examinations as often as the patient with poor plaque control, ongoing pathological wear or some other form of chronic dental disease. In this respect, the regular attender should be expected to make and honour a commitment to return for a dental examination after a specified period of time, either by obtaining an appointment for recall or by entering into a continuing care scheme arranged by their practitioner. A regularly attending patient may reasonably expect most of their treatment to be related to the maintenance of oral health, with the application of non-invasive forms of treatment, including, various preventive measures, advice and monitoring.

The pattern of provision of treatment for the regular attender may be based on responses to suggested preventive measures such as diet control, fluoride toothpaste use and plaque management. By these means, the prognosis of monitoring as opposed to intervention may be assessed. The ability to 'wait and see' may exist for the regular attender in contrast to the irregular attender. In this respect, it has been considered that the modern diagnostic approach is to answer the critical question, 'Is active caries present, and if so, at what rate is it progressing?' (Anusavice 1995) rather than 'Is there caries?'.

The role of monitoring

In patients who present with treatment needs but no acute problems, there are many advantages in the initial phase of treatment comprising largely of various forms of monitoring. Patients may be monitored as to their ability to maintain an acceptable level of oral hygiene, and an appropriate diet. Details of alcohol consumption and the patient's control or discontinuation of oral habits, smoking and other such activities, which may be regarded as indicators of poor oral health prognosis, are also of relevance when monitoring a patient. During the monitoring phase, initial management and treatment may be commenced. Aspects of the diagnosis may need to be deferred, depending upon clinical findings, such as the extent of caries, need for endodontic treatment, the rate of progression and periodicity of periodontal deterioration and wear. By these means, aspects of the patient's dental care may be evaluated and the various phases of treatment planned and provided in the form of a logical progression. Furthermore, diagnosis and treatment planning may continue throughout treatment, constantly changing to take account of the patients' problems and response to treatment. In this regard, contingency plans and options should be constantly re-evaluated as treatment progresses, possibly within the framework of a treatment flow chart. From the outset, however, the aims and objectives of treatment must be set and agreed with the patient.

1.2 ESTABLISHING THE PATIENT'S NEEDS

The importance of the initial interaction with a patient cannot be overstressed if the patient's dental needs are to be established. To facilitate history taking, it is necessary for the dentist to 'get to know' the patient and their expectations and aspirations. Readers are also referred to the section on felt and expressed needs as described in chapter 2, section 1.7.

Getting to know the patient

The initial interview with the patient should be conducted, wherever possible, in a relaxed environment away from the clinical situation, where the dentist and patient may discuss the patient's problems. Visual aids should be available. The approach and coordination of the dental team should inspire confidence in the patient, who should be aware of the confidentiality of all information given and recorded. A structured questionnaire may be used to assess or profile the patient's personality and level of dental anxiety (see Chapter 2: Assessment of Dental Anxiety). In addition, questionnaires identifying the following confounding factors may be of value:
- dental history,
- medical history,
- dietary preferences,
- oral function, and
- oral hygiene.

The patient's principal complaint and reason for attendance should be ascertained, including an understanding of the motivation, be it self motivation, peer pressure or pressure from friends, relation or partner. In this respect, it is essential that the patient appreciates the need for treatment, as misunderstandings can lead to difficulties in compliance, and may ultimately prejudice the success of treatment.

The examination

The examination of the patient must be holistic. The examination undertaken for the regular attender should be similar in detail and just as thorough as that undertaken for the irregularly attending patient, given that there may be a risk, in the regularly attending patient, of missing changes in their oral condition as a consequence of operator familiarity and complacence. Detailed recording of teeth and restorations present, caries, tooth wear, the periodontal condition, TMJ function and the condition of the mucosa is therefore of importance. In this respect, the use of a standardised examination in association with, for example, an Index of Oral Health (Burke and Wilson 1995) or an Oral Health Score (Chapter 2: Fig 2.8 on Assessment of Professional and Lay Perceptions or Need) may be of value in measuring the oral health status of the patient and comparing this with similar assessments at previous examinations. The availability of a questionnaire to be completed at each examination may also obviate the potential for problems to go undiagnosed. Such a questionnaire should encourage patients to discuss and describe their assessment (felt need) of the following:
- dental attractiveness (good/acceptable/unsightly)
- functional comfort (good/acceptable/cause for concern/poor)

- dental well-being (good/acceptable/cause for concern/poor)
- attitude to dentistry/the dentist (trusting/suspicious)
- ability to accept treatment (good/adequate/poor)

In addition, consideration should be given to the patient's economic situation, since a treatment plan must be tailored to the patient's ability to pay, and when the patient is covered by third-party insurance, the terms and conditions of the insurance cover must be taken into account. It may be argued that economic circumstances should not influence the development of an 'ideal' plan, and that the patient is the best judge of what can be afforded. Consideration of the cost of treatment, is however essential, if only to allow several alternatives at different levels of cost to be put to the patient. The cost-benefits of various treatments may also be discussed in the light of evidence-based research as to the effectiveness of particular forms of treatment. Accordingly, the provision of too simple or too complex a treatment plan based on incorrect assumptions about the patient's economic status will be avoided. Open, frank discussions about the cost of treatment should be encouraged and the treatment plan may be modified as a result.

Dietary analysis may be also appropriate to patients who, for example, have a present or past history of active caries or who have recently adopted unhealthy patterns of confectionery consumption. The results of these investigations should be retained in the patient's records for future reference. It may be necessary to examine the reasons for any shift in thinking or attitude if it becomes apparent that there has been a shift in the patient's behaviour – e.g. sucking mints as a smoking cessation aid.

An oral examination should aim to evaluate the overall oral health of the patient and should contain details of the following:

- caries activity,
- the adequacy of the patient's previous restorative care,
- the nature and extent of tooth wear,
- the adequacy of endodontic treatment,
- the health of the periodontal tissues,
- the adequacy of the occlusion,
- the health of the temporomandibular joint,
- patient comfort in function,
- dental appearance and attractiveness, and
- the health of the mucosa.

1.3 DECISIONS

Decisions to replace or to monitor restorations and root fillings, to treat or monitor caries and tooth wear, and to treat or monitor a periodontal condition should be made with regard to improvements which may be made to overall oral health. It may be argued, however, that the first decisions to be made should be those concerning active caries and progressive periodontal disease.

Caries management

The management of caries is dependent upon an assessment of the risk associated with leaving disease present; this, in turn, may be related to the overall level of oral health. The risk may be assessed more readily in the regularly attending patient than in the infrequent attender, given that the operator will have details of past disease experience, plaque control and patient motivation; past disease having been considered to be the most accurate predictor of risk (Pienihakkinen 1987). It has been considered by Kidd and Smith (1990) that caries risk assessment is notoriously difficult and that no one method has been developed to reliably predict caries activity in individuals. The extent of previous restorative work, extractions as a consequence of caries and the number of previous root canal treatments may be assessed during clinical examination and a retrospective review of the patient's notes, although such information may only be available for the regular attender. Nevertheless, the presence of active caries should alert the practitioner to the need to commence dietary analysis, preventive measures, and more frequent radiographic examinations of the regularly attending patient. The patient's medical and social history may also indicate a cause of increased caries incidence, such as the onset of Sjogren's disease or the prescription of medication which may result in reduced salivary flow. In this respect, a new direction in care may be indicated by the onset of systemic disease. The past fluoride experience of the patient, if known, may also be of relevance in deciding the treatment to be planned.

For diagnosis of caries, good lighting, dry clean teeth and a blunt probe are indicated (Kidd 1989), a blunt probe being considered appropriate given that probing with a sharp probe has been found to produce irreversible iatrogenic damage to occlusal fissures (Ekstrand *et al.* 1987). Following diagnosis, with consideration as to ways to shift the patient into a low risk category, the patient may be considered on a scale of high risk to low risk following analysis of the questionnaires completed at the initial interview. By so doing, initial lesions of caries which have not yet cavitated and not yet been diagnosed clinically or radiographically as being into dentine, may be treated using recalcification techniques in an attempt to delay further progression. The condition of the caries should be kept under regular review for patients who are prepared to attend at the required time intervals.

For the regularly attending patient, therefore, a decision should be made to resist the temptation to treat early caries, and monitor instead, having explained to the patient the rationale behind such a decision.

Periodontal assessment

Periodic assessments of the health of the periodontal tissues of a regularly attending patient are an integral aspect of continuing dental care. These may take the form of plaque scores, Basic Periodontal Examination (BPE) assessments and pocket depth measurements. In this respect, the routine use of a periodontal probe is an essential aspect of a routine dental evaluation. Any deterioration in periodontal condition, as evidenced by changes in assessments, should lead to further clinical and radiographical investigation, and intervention as necessary. Good health of the periodontal tissues is a prerequisite to achieving a satisfactory outcome in restorative care.

To replace or not to replace?

Many restorations last only short periods of time. Accordingly, assessment of the quality of existing restorations is an important aspect of the patient examination. Opportunities should be sought to maintain rather than replace existing restorations, as the life of amalgam restorations may be extended by supervising their aging process (Barbakow *et al.* 1988).

Restorations commonly fail in one of two ways, namely, new disease or technical failure. New disease may include new caries either around a restoration or at another site on the tooth, tooth wear, and pulpal pathology and restorations may also fail as a result of trauma. Technical failures include fracture of restorations, marginal breakdown, change in colour of tooth-coloured restorations and fracture of cusps adjacent to restorations, and may also include loss of the restoration because of inadequate retention. Defective contour, overhanging margins, discolouration and wear may be reasons for dentists to replace restorations.

Many modes of failure in restorations may be diagnosed in an objective manner, but marginal breakdown is a more subjective judgement which may or may not be a reason for replacement. Marginal deficiencies have been shown to be poorly correlated with the presence of active caries (Espelid and Tveit 1991), and it has been suggested that a restoration should be deemed to have failed if there is a 1 mm deep defect at its margin, or if dentine or base is exposed (Kidd *et al.* 1992).

In view of the poor correlation between caries and defective margins of restorations, the adoption of a conservative approach would appear prudent. This is applicable for, in particular, the regular attender in whom areas of doubtful marginal integrity around restorations may be monitored on a regular basis. Accordingly, the decision to maintain, replace or repair a restoration should be made in light of the patient's dental history. In this respect, Anusavice (1995) has considered that an assessment of the risk of caries and measurement of the rate of caries progression should be part of the decision-making process and has suggested that it is possible to compute the possible outcome. A conservative (non-intervention) approach should be adopted, given the lack of definitive guidelines and the poor correlation between defective margins and caries. Restorations should therefore be recontoured and refurbished or repaired wherever possible, and when a decision is made to modify and thereby preserve a restoration, the modified restoration should ideally be as good as when it was originally placed. If a decision is made to replace a restoration, it is essential that the cause of restoration failure is ascertained and that the design faults which led to failure of the restoration are recognised and not built into the new restoration. As in all healthcare provision, a preventative approach to patient management is preferable to a disease management approach. By so doing, the oral health of the patient should benefit and, in turn, the patient's well-being.

Patient awareness of dental aesthetics is increasing. Accordingly, some patients may request the replacement of satisfactory but unaesthetic restorations with tooth-coloured materials. In such cases, it is incumbent on the dentist to discuss any potential advantages and disadvantages of the tooth-coloured materials to be used.

In summary, in the light of current evidence, restorations should be refurbished or repaired wherever possible. In this respect, in the regularly attending patient, amalgam restorations should not be replaced solely because of marginal defects, except when the defects are very large. A similar philosophy may be applied to restorations of other materials. In such cases, an alternative approach is the localised repair, commencing cavity preparation in the area where caries has been diagnosed and deciding whether repair is viable once the caries has been removed.

Assessment of wear

Assessment of tooth substance loss (TSL) forms an important part of the assessment of the continuing oral health of a patient. Treatment may be indicated only in cases in which the overall oral health is prejudiced, for factors such as loss of function, discomfort, or poor aesthetics (as perceived by the patient), having first made a decision whether the tooth surface loss is physiological or pathological. Treatment may be necessary to reduce sensitivity, protect the teeth from further wear and to restore the teeth to proper form and function. To assess the progression of wear, it may be necessary to obtain serial study casts and photographic records. (See also Section 6.6, Chapter 4.)

The dental practitioner may be the first to diagnose problems such as bulimia, with wear normally occurring principally on the palatal aspect of upper teeth and on the occlusal aspect of molar teeth. The clinician must be in a position to recognise these signs of disease and institute treatment in conjunction with other healthcare workers.

Assessment of endodontic treatment

The health of the periapical tissues of endodontically treated teeth may be assessed by absence of pain, swelling and other symptoms, a sinus tract, loss of function and radiographic evidence of a normal periodontal ligament around the root. Root canal treatment may not be considered a success if radiographic examination indicates that a lesion is apparently unchanged or has only diminished in size. In such situations, the European Society for Endodontology (1994) advises that the lesion be monitored until it resolves or for a period of four years. If, after four years, resolution has not occurred, the root canal treatment should be considered a failure, with further treatment by conventional retreatment, endodontic surgery or extraction being indicated. The regularly attending patient may therefore expect monitoring of endodontic treatment until the success or failure of such treatment is ascertained. It may, however, be anticipated that practitioners may prefer non-intervention and radiographic monitoring to extraction.

1.4 PRIORITIES IN TREATMENT

Following observation and analysis of a patient's problems, treatment should be prioritised. Complex problems should be divided into component elements which are relatively easy to resolve or which facilitate understanding of the nature and complexity of the underlying problem (Verdonschot 1984).

Decisions may be made on each particular problem using a decision-tree approach (Hall *et al.* 1994). Priority should be given to those problems of an urgent or emergency nature or those which pose a threat to the patient's general health, followed by the removal and control of pathological factors, restoration, maintenance and recall. Accordingly, in considering the patient's treatment priorities, treatments which contribute to oral and general health may be considered a priority following pain relief.

The following may be considered to be a basis for fulfilling these criteria, although any treatment plan should be capable of being amended following monitoring or changes in prognosis following investigation.

(i) Diagnosis and control of pain

The clinician should initially attend to the complaint which has led to the patient's attendance, although acute problems cannot always be solved immediately. Failure to diagnose and control pain may lead to poor patient compliance.

(ii) Patient education

Educating patients with regard to the causes, nature and prognosis of dental disease should be commenced early during treatment, and should be reinforced throughout treatment (see also Section 2.0 of this chapter, Promoting Oral Health in Primary Dental Care). Details of, for example, toothbrushing frequency and techniques, control of sugar intake, should be included. Patient instruction with regard to the mode of action of fluoride may also be of value. Practice information leaflets may be useful.

(iii) Periodontal care

In cases in which the periodontal status is compromised, it may be necessary to initiate a course of simple periodontal therapy and review the outcome, before finalising a plan of definitive treatment. Occlusal adjustments should, where indicated, be carried out at this stage to eliminate gross interferences and control aggravating factors; splint therapy should be contemplated as a means to obtain control of the deranged occlusion. More than six months may be required before the effectiveness of initial periodontal therapy may be apparent.

(iv) Control of caries activity

Active caries should be controlled before considering definitive treatment. In this respect, manufacturers have introduced lactic acid indicator swabs and saliva buffering and flow tests, both of which help display potential caries activity to patients.

As mentioned previously, diet diaries must be used to assess and analyse the patient's diet. Dietary counselling may help the patient control their cariogenic dietary habits. Fluoride in the form of toothpastes, daily and weekly mouthwashes and supplements should be instituted to prevent further episodes of dental caries. Investigation and treatment of extensive caries may assist in determining the need for endodontic therapy, with the associated implications of cost and time. In the initial treatment of caries, glass polyalkenoate (ionomer) cements offer benefits such as ease of use and fluoride release, and may therefore be used as interim restorations.

(v) Oral surgery

The extraction of asymptomatic teeth considered to be either unrestorable, in an abnormal position or of poor prognosis from the periodontal viewpoint, should be carried out once the patient's confidence permits consideration of this phase of treatment. This phase may also include removal of high fraenal attachments, modification of ridge forms etc.

(vi) Restoration of primary caries

When the clinician considers that primary caries requires operative intervention, a decision must be reached regarding the most suitable management of the lesion. It is desirable that a restoration which limits the need to remove sound tooth tissue is chosen, provided that such an approach is compatible with an acceptable prognosis.

(vii) Endodontic treatment

Teeth of functional and cosmetic importance which are considered or found to be non-vital or for which radiographic examination suggests that pulpal exposure is inevitable, should be treated by endodontic therapy at an early stage. It should first be ascertained, however, that restoration of the crown of the tooth to be root-treated is feasible. Elective endodontic therapy may also be appropriate in some cases, for example where teeth are considered suitable as overdenture abutments.

Core build-ups should be completed at this stage, both on vital teeth destined to be crowned, and on non-vital teeth prior to endodontic treatment, in order to facilitate moisture control and the application of rubber dam.

(viii) Orthodontic treatment

Where a malocclusion is present, or overcrowding of teeth is either aesthetically or functionally undesirable, an orthodontic opinion should be sought once periodontal therapy has been successfully completed and caries has been controlled. It may be appropriate to leave indirect restorations until orthodontic treatment has been completed, although the cores for these restorations should be placed. In anterior teeth, even if crowns are planned as the long term restoration, acid-etch retained restorations should be placed until the final tooth position has been achieved.

(ix) Replacement or maintenance of existing restorations

Restorations may be replaced or maintained according to the criteria discussed above. Decisions to leave a suspect restoration should be substantiated, and in such cases it is important to advise the patient of the decision to moni-tor such suspect restorations. Additionally, premolar and permanent molar teeth which have been successfully root filled should be considered for restoration by cusp protecting restorations.

The cost of restoration modification and repair should normally be substantially less than the cost of renewal, and it may be possible to achieve either a satisfactory long term result or to use the restoration as a long term temporary until such time as the patient can justify the cost of replacement.

(x) Crowns

The provision of indirect restorations is normally appropriate only for patients in whom a good response has been achieved following the periodon-tal and caries control phases of treatment, as failure to achieve success in these phases will normally prejudice the longevity of the crowns, bridges etc. Discussion with the patient may assist in determining the type of restoration to be provided, for example, full or three-quarter coverage, using gold or porcelain. Consideration of the type of temporary restoration to be provided is also an important element of treatment planning, as is the recognition of the need for the provision of occlusal rims for occlusal registration. Furthermore, in planning more advanced and, in particular, extensive courses of treatment, consideration must be given as to whether to adopt a conformative or reorganised approach to the patient's occlusion.

(xi) Management of edentulous spaces

Restoration of edentulous spaces demands considerable commitment from a patient, in particular, when the space is to be restored with a removable pros-thesis. The provision of such an appliance is therefore contraindicated unless the patient is aware of the potential value of the prosthesis and the draw-backs associated with its use. This may not present a problem when there is a demonstrable aesthetic advantage from the prosthesis. By contrast, where the value is purely functional, the advantages associated with the provision of the prosthesis will require careful explanation if patient acceptance is to be achieved. Furthermore, the provision of a removable partial denture should be considered carefully from the aspect of function, given that clinical investi-gations among subjects with shortened dental arches have shown that there is sufficient adaptive capacity to maintain oral function when only four occlusal units are left (Kayser *et al.* 1987). Treatment with removable partial dentures may also produce unfavourable conditions for the remaining denti-tion. Consequently, the benefits of providing such an appliance should be carefully weighed against the potential disadvantages. In shortened dental arches in which anterior crowns are to be provided, the need for provision of posterior support should be given careful consideration, given that the prognosis of the anterior crowns may be reduced if posterior occlusal support is not provided. Nevertheless, it is not always necessary to extend a free-end removable partial denture to the full extent of an arch.

For patients for whom a prosthesis is required, radiographs should be available of all abutment teeth, which should also be tested for vitality. Assessments of articulated study casts and associated occlusal investigations should also be completed at an early stage.

(xii) Maintenance

Success or failure of treatment is dependent on correct planning and the provision of high quality care, together with the institution of an effective maintenance regime. Decisions should be made regarding the frequency of recall required, depending on the special needs of each patient. Notes should be made concerning the specific areas which may require special attention, together with potential measures which may be necessary. It is at this stage that the need for regular attendance should be reinforced with the irregular attender.

(xiii) Audit

Evaluation of the success of treatment and its planning should be an integral part of self-assessment, peer review and clinical audit, with the clinician being prepared to alter the approach if it becomes apparent that successful results are not being achieved. This may also form the basis of clinical governance.

1.5 PROBLEM SOLVING

The adoption of a problem-oriented approach in patient assessment and treatment planning has been suggested by Kayser *et al.* (1988), for at least partially dentate adult dental patients. These workers suggest that the substantial amount of information collected during the initial assessment and examination of a patient should be 'funnelled' until only the core information remains. By completing an inventory of all the patient's dental problems, it is suggested that these may then be critically appraised to determine whether they are relevant to the patient's oral health or for the maintenance of the dentition. Accordingly, it is suggested that treatment planning should be based on the functional requirements of the patient. For example, if a patient complains of an inability to chew, s/he should be encouraged to demonstrate the problem to the dentist who, in turn, should arguably only treat or replace the teeth giving rise to the patient's problems, given that it has been shown that patients may maintain adequate dental function with shortened dental arches. Such an approach, which it is suggested will increasingly find application in the management of adult patients, may extend over a number of visits, but will enable the clinician to diagnose the patient's problems and determine the treatment priorities in the context of the patient's expectations. Once the patient's treatment priorities have been determined, treatment may be organised in phases as described above.

A problem-solving approach was also described by Verdonschot in 1984. He reviewed the literature to ascertain the sequence in which dental problems had been treated, finding that, of the four authors examined, all gave priority to complaints and emergencies. One author, Balshi (1980), listed acute pathology, caries and plaque control, endodontics, establishment of vertical dimension, orthodontics, provisional restorations and oral surgical procedures in the first phase of treatment. Based on his review, Verdonschot (1984) classified problems according to the urgency with which they should be solved, as follows:

- immediate problems – those affecting general health, complaints and emergencies.
- microbial problems – caries, periodontitis, periapical problems and endodontic problems.
- reconstructive problems – chronic periodontitis, occlusal problems, articulation problems, orthodontic problems, restoration of tooth resistance to functional load.
- maintenance problems – remotivation, adjustment and review.

In conclusion, a major objective of oral health education should be to create and reinforce social expectations related to health, with patients appreciating the need to adopt and sustain routines of behaviour which will maintain health by the prevention of disease. In this way, it is hoped to change the irregular attender to a regular attender by means of a treatment plan which suits the patient.

Many alternative strategies typically exist for patients with extensive treatment needs. Restoration of posterior occlusal support prior to the restoration of dental appearance by the restoration of the anterior teeth is one approach. Alternatively, the early achievement of a cosmetic improvement may bring improvements in oral hygiene, motivation and dental awareness in patients in whom this is lacking, although there may then be a risk that the patient may not return for the functional improvements which would be achieved by restoration of the posterior dentition. Several treatment modalities may run concurrently, for example, periodontal therapy and caries management. In all cases, the temptation to overtreat should be resisted, and a problem-oriented approach adopted. It would therefore appear reasonable to determine and treat the patient's immediate problems, in particular, those which may affect general health.

Priorities identified by the dentist may differ from those perceived by the patient if the initial interview with the patient does not properly identify the patient's expectations. Treatment planning should be based on evidence-based research, while the patient's priorities may be altogether more subjective. The reconciliation of these potentially different points of view is necessary if a treatment plan is to succeed, but such an approach may require considerable skill in patient management.

The approach which has been presented allows the progress of different treatment modalities in a logical manner, preceded by relief of pain carried out within an overall treatment strategy. Many more patients are now regular dental attenders than in the past and should therefore be assessed in terms of quality of oral health rather than in terms of disease levels – a traditional approach now appropriate only to the irregular attender. The dental health-care worker must adopt a mindset towards the maintenance of oral health rather than constantly reacting to disease.

In all cases, before proceeding with treatment, the patient's consent (either written or implied) to treatment must be obtained.

No two patients are the same, and for any one patient many potential strategies for treatment planning are generally appropriate. These strategies may be influenced by a large variety of patient and dentist related factors. Nevertheless, correct diagnosis and an effective assessment of the patient's expectations should be combined to provide an overall, long term, treatment philosophy, ultimately producing a treatment plan and order of treatment with which both operator and patient feel comfortable. Above all else, the treatment must be justifiable and for the long term benefit of the patient. Treatment priorities are summarised in Table 4.1.

2.0 PROMOTING ORAL HEALTH IN PRIMARY DENTAL CARE

The practice of dentistry is composed of two distinct philosophies – the restorative philosophy and the preventive philosophy. These are intertwined and reflect the diversity of primary dental care. The restorative philosophy provides the dentist with his livelihood, whereas the preventive philosophy supports, underpins and sustains all the restorative care provided for the patient. Incorporating a preventive philosophy into primary dental care allows the dentist and his team to inculcate the practice with a health promotion attitude that encourages and empowers patients to seize control of their own oral health.

The view that primary health care should be of a preventive orientation is not new, as highlighted by the World Health Organisation (WHO 1978).

Table 4.1 Treatment priorities to be considered

Diagnosis and control of pain

Patient education

toothbrushing frequency and techniques

control of sucrose intake

build patient confidence

Initial Periodontal therapy

simple periodontal therapy

review progress

occlusal adjustments-eliminate gross interferences

splint therapy

more complex therapy

Control of caries activity

active caries control before considering definitive treatment. Investigation/treatment
    of extensive carious lesions

diet history

diet analysis and counselling

fluoride toothpaste

fluoride supplements

fluoride mouthwashes

Oral Surgery

removal of unrestorable teeth, or those of poor periodontal prognosis (when patient
    confidence has increased)

removal of high fraenal attachments

modification of ridge forms

Restoration of primary carious lesions

Endodontic treatment

non-vital teeth or where pulpal exposure is inevitable, provided that restoration of the
    crown of the tooth is feasible

elective endodontic therapy appropriate in some cases, for overdenture abutments.

core build-ups completed at this stage

Orthodontic treatment

malocclusion

overcrowding which is aesthetically or functionally undesirable

leave indirect restorations until orthodontic treatment has been completed

Replacement of existing restorations

root-filled premolar/molar teeth replaced by cusp protecting restorations

replace other restorations when recurrent caries or fracture

Maintenance of existing restorations

evaluate quality of existing restoration

leave, replace or modify the restoration in accordance with patient's dental history,
    level of dental awareness and potential for future attendance

(Continued)

Table 4.1 (continued) Treatment priorities to be considered

polish existing composite restorations to remove marginal staining
polish amalgam restoration margins if marginal defects present
recontour and remove marginal overhangs
adjust areas of hyperocclusion
restore aesthetically poor crown margins

Crowns
appropriate for patients with good response to periodontal and caries control phases
consider type of restoration, e.g. full or three-quarter coverage, gold or porcelain,
   occlusal coverage by porcelain
consider type of temporary restoration
recognition need for occlusal rims

Management of edentulous spaces
assess radiographs of abutment teeth
assess study casts
provide appliance only where patient is aware of its value
provide posterior support or improve aesthetics.

Maintenance treatment
Audit
evaluate success of treatment and planning

The WHO (1978) not only perceived primary health care as accessible, appropriate, acceptable, available and affordable to communities at every stage of their development; but also recognised the importance of appropriate health care technology and emphasised the prevention of disease (Maybela and Freeman 1985).

The responsibility for the shift from traditional concepts of primary care to those envisaged by WHO (1978) lie with policy makers. It may be proposed that the responsibility for the shift from restorative to preventive philosophy rests with the dentist. S/he will set the parameters, employ the staff and provide the physical environment (the preventive dental unit) in which the oral health promotion aspects of his/her practice will be accessible, available and affordable to all the patients under his/her care. This means that the dentist must have prior knowledge of the determinants of health behaviours and what constitutes health promotion in contrast to health education.

The skills necessary to promote oral health in the general practice setting include formulating practice and putting oral health promotion on the practice agenda. The dentist must be able to roll out the practice policy, in terms of the plans for action to the dental team so that they may be empowered with an understanding of the principles and aims of health promotion and

how these may be applied to primary dental care. The dental team's awareness of the models of health behaviour together with an appreciation of the difficulties people experience when trying to change their habits, will provide a working environment conducive to the promotion of oral health. In addition, the dentist must have the skills to plan, manage and evaluate oral health promotion in the practice. The dentist must also possess the necessary finance, knowledge of health promotion/education/behaviour, appropriate staff, health education aids and baseline data from which evaluations may be made.

The movement from restorative to preventive philosophy can therefore be thought of as a series of steps (fig. 4.1). The first step is to formulate the practice policy in terms of broad strategic aims which define health promotion as well as specific health education aims that characterise the type of health education that will be conducted within the practice setting. The second step is to plan the delivery of the oral health promotion. This will include financial implications for the practice (affordability), where the oral health promotion will be conducted (accessibility, acceptable), who will deliver the health education (availability, acceptable) and what resources will be needed (appropriate, availability). The third step is the management of the preventive dental unit, the methods used to promote oral health and

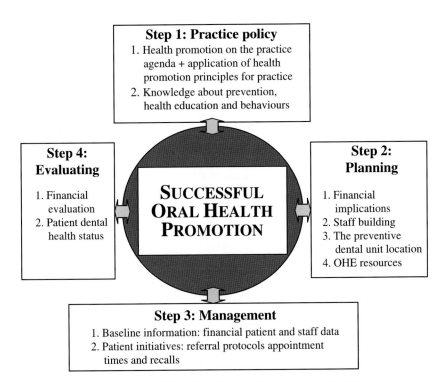

Figure 4.1 Actions for successful oral health promotion in primary dental care.

collection of baseline data. The final step is evaluation of the programme. This integrated approach will permit the dentist and his/her team to create an atmosphere in which prevention underpins the practice of dentistry and with this shift in emphasis the dental practice changes its guise within an 'oral health promoting practice' framework .

2.1 STEP 1 DEVELOPING PRACTICE POLICY

Health promotion

Health promotion is said to be the advancement of health by changing the environment and giving people the ability to seize control of their health. Within the health promotion scenario the individuals' ability to change their health behaviour is subsumed within a healthy environment which allows people to make the 'healthy choice the easy choice'. The reasoning for the need to encourage shifts from less healthy to more healthy environments is related to the fact that the determinants of health are first environmental and secondly, behavioural.

McKeown's (1979) work showed that the environmental determinants of health were nutrition, sanitation, housing, immunisation and therapeutics, and limitation of the family size. Behavioural determinants were related to lifestyle and health behaviours – for example a diet high in fats, tobacco smoking and a sedentary lifestyle were implicated in cardio-vascular disease. However, these determinants did not exist in isolation and were operative within the social milieu. Factors connected with socio-economic status, relative wealth, relative poverty and level of education attained had all been shown to intensify unhealthy behaviours resulting in health inequalities. The difficulty that existed was that health education, per se, rather than reducing health inequalities between socio-economic groups sustained them with ever increasing health divisions being observed within society. The requirement to find a means by which health inequalities could be addressed resulted in a shift from health education to health promotion as the cornerstone of strategies to improve the health of a population.

The awareness that environmental, behavioural and social measures were important resulted in the World Health Organisation (1981) statement that:

> 'all people in all countries should have at least such a level of health that they are capable of working productively and of participating actively in the social life of the community in which they live'.

Three health goals were identified:
(i) the promotion of life-styles conducive to health; for example enabling people to take control over their lifestyles, defining priority policies for action, for example nutrition (nutrition and dental caries), tobacco (smoking cessation in primary dental care) and policies concerned with the environment

(ii) prevention of preventable conditions (for example, dental caries)

(iii) rehabilitation and health services (for example, primary dental care).

Strategic aims of health promotion (the Ottawa Charter WHO 1986)

In 1986 the WHO launched the Ottawa Charter. It provided a basis for policy and strategy with respect to health promotion within the wider environment and within primary health care. The five principles of health promotion reflected the need to address both the environmental and behavioural determinants of health. Some of the principles, therefore, appear not to be directly applicable to primary dental care but an appreciation of them will furnish the dentist with preventive attitude for his/her practice (Table 4.2). The final principle illustrates the requirement of those in dental practice to have an awareness and to adopt a preventive attitude with regard to the promotion of health within primary care. Working in this way will enable the dental team to develop appropriate practice-based health education strategies (Principles 2 and 3) to assist their patients in the development of their own personal, health skills.

Strategies to change the principles of health promotion into policy have been suggested (WHO 1986). These are intended for the wider political arena. However, they are applicable for the dental practice that intends to adopt the oral health promotion agenda. Using the framework suggested by WHO (1986) the practitioner may stipulate practice policy and the oral health promotion agenda. This will result in a series of broad aims that may be applied and incorporated into the practice. Parallels between policy issues for the promotion of health in general and the broad aims for oral health as determined

---

Table 4.2 The Ottawa Charter's Principles of Health Promotion

The Principles of Health Promotion (WHO 1986)

1. Health promotion actively involves the population in the setting of everyday life rather than focusing on people who are at risk for specific conditions and in contact with medical services (**e.g. water fluoridation**).
2. Health promotion is directed towards action on the causes of ill health (**e.g. oral health education on a one-to-one basis**)
3. Health promotion uses many different approaches which combine to improve health (**e.g. smoking cessation programmes in primary dental care**).
4. Health promotion depends particularly on public participation
5. Health professionals – especially those in **primary health care** – have an important part to play in nurturing health promotion and enabling it to take place (**e.g. provision of material, staff and time resources for oral health promotion**).

by the dentist exist – building healthy 'practice' policies, for instance, are analogous to the building of public policies for health. Creating a supportive environment for oral health within the practice setting is equivalent to the creation of supportive environments for general health. Forging methodologies which strengthen the patients' determination to achieve their negotiated oral health goals may be thought of in the same terms as strengthening community action. In addition, the strengthening of the dental team's resolve to put oral health promotion on the agenda potentiates the assimilation of health promotion concepts into practice life. The development of personal skills (knowledge and health actions) may be incorporated into the primary dental care environment. Patients together with the dental team will be empowered with oral health knowledge and will be aware of the necessary personal [health] skills (e.g. inter-dental cleaning techniques) needed to support and maintain oral health.

The framework of principles and strategic aims, contained within Ottawa Charter (WHO 1986), provides the dentist with a series of broad aims and objectives by which restorative orientated practice may be modified into a more preventive practice (Table 4.3). The practice policy is evidence based (health promotion principles) and the aims providing the dentist with his/her practice agenda. Together the practice policy and agenda allow the dental team to take their first steps on the pathway to successful oral health promotion in primary dental care.

Health education, health behaviours, and preventive dentistry

A knowledge and understanding of health education, health behaviours and how these integrated with preventive dentistry is the next stage in formulating practice policy. This section will not examine the scientific basis of dental health education (Levine 1996) but will provide examples of models of health education and behaviour. The preferred model(s) of health education and behaviour will set the agenda for the manner and delivery of the oral health message and it is at this point that the dentist will clarify and focus the aims and objectives that will be appropriate for his practice needs.

(i) Models of health education
The dentist in formulating his/her practice policy, must decide what is his/her specific aim in terms of oral health outcome for his/her patients. This is determined by the characteristics of the surrounding environment in terms of the psychosocial profile, the prevalence of oral disease, and the desired oral health outcome deemed appropriate for the practice. There are various models of health education (Table 4.4) which range from clinical techniques to prevent disease ('the medical model') to those which allow the patient to set the health agenda ('client-centred model'). The difficulty in choosing any one

Table 4.3 The aims of health promotion and their application to primary dental care

Health promotion aims (Ottawa Charter: WHO 1986)	Application of health promotion aims for Primary Dental Care
1. Build public policies which support health Health becomes an item on the agenda of all policy makers, requires governmental and organisational action.	1. Build practice policies which support oral health Oral health promotion is on the practice agenda. Facilities, staff and resources are available to support oral health promotion within the practice setting
2. Create supportive environments for health Health promotion must create living and working conditions that are safe, stimulating, satisfying and enjoyable.	2. Create supportive environments for oral health The practice must be an environment in which oral health promotion is a priority. The conditions are such that it promotes oral health, e.g. a sugar-free zone; a smoke-free zone
3. Strengthen community action Health promotion works by giving people control over their own initiatives and actions. It requires health professionals to work for and with communities (rather than on them).	3. Strengthen practice action By negotiating oral health goals with patients and giving them control over their own oral health initiatives and actions. Dental health professionals to work with patients recognizing their felt and expressed needs rather than imposing their owns views (normative need) upon patients.
4. Develop personal skills Health promotion supports personal and social development by providing information, health education, and helping people to develop skills necessary to make healthy choices.	4. Develop personal oral health skills Oral health promotion supports the patient's personal and social development by providing health information and helping them to develop skills necessary for oral health (e.g. flossing techniques)
5. Re-orientate health services The responsibility for health promotion in health services is a shared responsibility for all individuals, community groups, health professionals and governments. They must work together towards a health care system which contributes to the pursuit of health.	5. Re-orientate dental health services The responsibility for oral health promotion in the practice is a shared responsibility between patients, nurses, receptionists, hygienists and dentists. The practice must be responsive to the patients' needs and work to develop a practice which contributes to the promotion of oral health.

Table 4.4 Five models of health education: applications for primary dental care

Model of health education	Aim	Health education/promotion activity	Examples for primary dental care
Medical model	To be free from disease and disability	Clinical preventive techniques to prevent disease	Fissure sealants, scale and polish, fluoride treatments
Education model	To provide health knowledge and understanding, health decisions are made and acted upon	Health education given together with an exploration of values and attitudes. Developing skills for healthier living	Smoking cessation programme in dental practice
Behaviour change model	To change of health behaviours to improve health	Assisting attitude and behaviour changes to encourage shifts from unhealthy to healthier lifestyles and behaviours	One-to-one dental health education at the chair-side on dietary advice for prevention of dental caries
Client-centred model	To negotiate health goals from the patient's perspective	Patients set the agenda and decide which health issues should be discussed. Patients empowered to negotiate their identified health goals	Negotiation of oral health goals to assist adolescents to reduce consumption of acidic drinks
Societal change model	To change physical and social environments to enable people to have healthier lifestyles	Political and social action to change physical/social environment	Fluoridation of the water

model over another is, that at any time, one model may be more appropriate than another for a particular patient. This has some importance, as within any practice population there will be healthy patients, patients who are at risk, patients who are suffering and patients who are recovering. Each group of patients will require different health education inputs and this has been described in terms of primary, secondary and tertiary prevention (Table 4.5). The adolescent with rampant caries will have different oral health education needs (tertiary prevention) than the adult patient who is trying to stop smoking (secondary prevention) or who requires oral hygiene instruction (primary prevention).

It is therefore necessary to remain flexible when formulating practice policy. In some situations the most suitable model may be the medical model as it provides a rationale for the use of fissure sealants, in children. Smoking cessation programmes based in dental practice raise awareness ('educational model') and have been shown to be a decisive element in assisting patients to stop smoking. In the tertiary prevention scenario, adults with destructive bone loss may be helped to improve their periodontal health by using a patient-centred approach ('client-centred model').

Irrespective of which health education model is used it is necessary that practice policy reflects that health education requirements vary between patients within a practice population and should be responsive to the patients' preventive needs throughout the life course.

(ii) Models of health behaviour

Models of health behaviour have been developed to increase the understanding of why some people adopt certain habits, why some are able to change from less healthy to more healthy behaviours and why others are resistant to change. There are various approaches to health education and these are reflected in the models of health education. These approaches include providing information (the Health Belief Model) to those who help patients set their own agenda (Motivational Interviewing) to change their health behaviours (Stages of Change Model).

Table 4.5 Health education requirements for different patient groups

Patient Group	Type of prevention	Health education
Healthy Average Risk	Primary prevention	Information on health threats
High Risk	Secondary prevention	Behaviour change required
Ill	Tertiary prevention	Recognise symptoms, take action and accept cure
Cured	Tertiary prevention	Follow rehabilitation programme

The health belief model (HBM)

A well-known cognitive model of health behaviour is the HBM (Rosenstock 1974). The HBM (fig. 4.2) proposes that health behaviour is dependent on:

- the perceived susceptibility to an illness
- the perceived severity of the illness
- the perceived threat of the illness
- if the benefits outweigh the barriers of taking action then behaviour change will occur

There were problems with the HBM as it tended to ignore the importance of demographic and cultural influences upon health. These were believed to be of secondary importance and so the model had the propensity to explain little of the behaviour under study. Consequently many of the attitudes associated

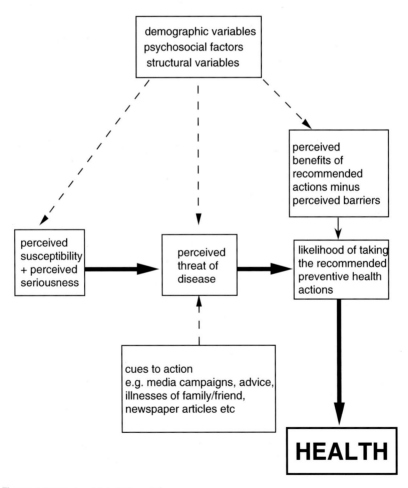

Figure 4.2 The health belief model.

with the behaviour remained hidden and the model fell out of favour. Modifications to the model have been made and these include:

- cues for action in the form of health information (e.g. media campaigns, newspaper articles) to motivate patients
- the influence of demographic, psychosocial factors and structural factors (fig. 4.3)

In the HBM, patients' compliance with advice on oral health care is assumed to be dependent upon perceived susceptibility, the potential severity of the condition and the costs of making the changes. Health education associated with the HBM is therefore, information based. People are informed of the threat and severity of diseases in order to help them accept and maintain healthier lifestyles.

Motivational interviewing and the stages of change model

Motivational interviewing and use of the stages of change model represent two other approaches to health education – namely agenda setting and empowerment and support. Bringing about lasting and effective changes

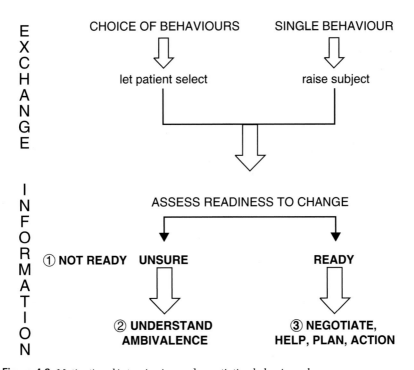

Figure 4.3 Motivational interviewing and negotiating behaviour change.

in health behaviours means assisting patients to explore dental health attitudes, discover their health values and encourage them to identify their own dental health agenda. This involves the dentist providing support for the patient. A number of principles of good practice have been identified. These are:
- respecting the patients' autonomy and that their choices are important
- readiness to change must be taken into account
- ambivalence is common and reasons for it need to be explored and understood
- target/goals should be identified by the patients
- you provide information and support
- the patient is the decision-maker and selects the behaviour(s) to be changed.

Motivational interviewing

In order to assist the patient in setting their own health agenda, motivational interviewing embraces the idea that it is the patients' degree of ambivalence or readiness to change which is the key to success. It is the assessment of the ambivalence or 'readiness to change' that is the essence of motivational interviewing (Rollnick *et al.* 1993) (fig. 4.3). Readiness to change is assessed using readiness to change rulers or agenda setting charts. It is essential, therefore, that patients are involved in identifying their degree of ambivalence and the behaviours to be modified. There are 3 possible outcomes of motivational interviewing:
① **The patient is not ready:** this must be accepted and the dentist must wait.
② **The patient is ambivalent:** the indecision of the patient must be acknowledged and the dentist must try to understand the patient's resistances.
③ **The patient is ready:** the health behaviours identified and health goals negotiated.

The stages of change model

The Stages of Change Model (Prochaska and DiClemente 1986) provides the next stage in supporting the patient to change their oral health behaviours. This model acknowledges that behaviour change is a complex process and is dependent on the patients' degree of ambivalence. The role of the dentist is to identify the patient's state of readiness and provide help and support to enable them to change from less healthy to more healthy actions. In this model, change is seen as a process, which has 5 interlinking stages (fig. 4.4):
① **Precontemplation:** the patient moves from unawareness to awareness and the need to change. The discussion of the benefits ('the pros') and the barriers ('the cons') provides the basis of the precontemplation stage. Interventions used include providing patients with health information and discovering lifestyle problems which might act as barriers to progressing to the next stage.

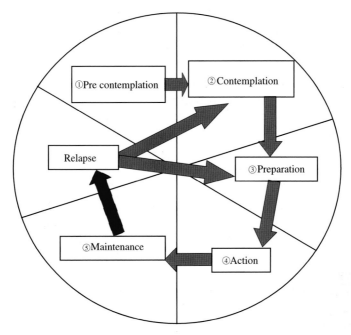

Figure 4.4 The Stages of Change Model.

② **Contemplation:** patients are weighing up the benefits ('the pros') against the barriers ('the cons') of changing their health behaviours. They are not yet ready to change and some patients get stuck in the contemplation stage and become 'chronic contemplators'. 'Chronic contemplators' should be seen on a regular basis as their indecision reflects their ambivalence.

③ **Preparation** can take a long time. It is essential for chronic contemplators as preparation time reduces ambivalence while improving self-awareness and self-image. The dentist's role is to provide patients with information and to assist them to think about their feelings about changing.

④ and ⑤ **Action and Maintenance:** these phases reflect the resolution of ambivalence. The pros of changing outweigh the cons. During the action phase the dentist usually works with the patients to help them identify realistic goals. In maintenance the interventions are shorter, more intensive and more participative to support patients maintain their newly acquired behaviours.

Relapse occurs when unhealthy behaviours are reinstated. This is common and provides time for re-negotiation of health goals. Relapse allows patient and health professional to recognise that what has been achieved and what will be achieved again. The dentist at relapse must be supportive and re-negotiate more realistic and achievable goals to help the patient. Patients usually do not return to precontemplation but may return to the contemplation stage and progress quickly through preparation to action.

In developing practice policy with regard to promoting oral health the dentist must be aware of the principles of health promotion, the various models of health behaviour and approaches to health education. This will provide the knowledge base from which planning of the preventive dental unit can be launched.

2.2 PLANNING THE PREVENTIVE DENTAL UNIT (PDU)

The next step is planning the PDU. This is an important part of the planning cycle as with careful preparation the PDU can be evaluated and modified in accordance with the changing needs of the practice. Benefits to the practice in terms of improved financial health, a more cohesive dental team and healthier patients must be given due consideration. In the Mentadent programme entitled 'profitable preventive practice' goal setting was perceived as a central part of the overall planning exercise. They suggested that the practitioner answer three questions, as part of the goal setting exercise:

1. Where is the practice now?	2. Where should we be?	3. How can we get there?
• *Patterns of prevention* not offering more prevention	• *Patterns of prevention* offer patients prevention	• *Patterns of prevention* employ hygienist, OHE
• *Premises* old fashioned image limited space	• *Premises* room for PDU modern image	• *Premises* extend premises to set up a PDU **OR** look for other premises

The planning stage includes goal setting, an assessment of the financial implications of setting up and running a PDU (equipment, staff, costs of training and oral health education resources); the need to instill a preventive philosophy in the dental team members; the location, design and layout and the type of oral health education aids to be available for the unit.

Financial implications: equipment and staff

Preventive technologies (clinical and health education interventions) in general practice has been suggested as a means of providing cost-effective prevention (Holloway *et al.* 1997). Details about the financial aspects of running a successful PDU are therefore essential and so as part of the planning process it is necessary to compile a business plan. The business plan should be clear, realistic and based upon the practice accounts together with details of additional financial expenditure (staff, premises, equipment, fixtures and fittings) to allow for successful oral health promotion in the practice setting.

The dentist must decide on whether to buy (lease purchase or hire-purchase) or lease equipment for the preventive dental unit. Both means of purchasing equipment will have implications for cash flow and budgeting within the practice. Leasing equipment helps with budgeting as the fixed monthly rental costs can be calculated into the practice's monthly expenditure and the rental may be tax deductible. At the end of the leasing period the equipment may be bought, upgraded or traded in for a newer model. The benefits of hire-purchase include tax relief on the bank loan and at the end of the loan period the equipment is owned outright.

The decision, with regard to which member(s) of the dental team will provide the oral health promotion, is an important issue, as this will have financial implications for the practice. Usually the choice is between the dental hygienist and a dental nurse who has been trained as a dental health educator. There are financial advantages and disadvantages with regard to choosing a hygienist rather than a dental health educator (Table 4.6). However, the decision on whom to employ must include the individual's knowledge and principles of oral health promotion, their ability to communicate effectively and to be able to undertake clinical preventive techniques (Table 4.6). This may result in further expense for the dental practice if the person chosen requires further training in the area of oral health promotion – for instance a dental nurse undertaking the post qualification course in 'oral health education'. The combination of all the above, together with an assessment of the cash flow and budgeting requirements of the practice will dictate the choice of a particular individual for the position within the PDU.

Team building

As mentioned elsewhere (see Chapter 3 and Section 1 The Dental Team) it is essential to have regular practice meetings. This allows team members to come to a collective decision as to who will take over the day-to-day management of the PDU. It will also allow team members to voice concerns and anxieties about the PDU, to understand the need for the PDU and to provide an arena for ideas for the development of the unit to be discussed. Issues relating to the targeting of specific patient groups can be aired at meetings. Promotional health education campaigns (e.g. 'No Smoking Day', 'Smile Week'), can be discussed and open days for the practice or family packages can be arranged. Using regular practice meetings will allow a cohesive approach to

Table 4.6 Personnel for the oral health promoting practice: financial implications

Personnel	The dentist	Dental hygienist	Dental health educator
Advantages	1. Sets the oral health promotion agenda;	1. Knows the theory and principles for practice;	1. Knows the theory and principles for practice;
	2. Knows the theory and principles for practice;	2. Good communicator;	2. Effective OHE communicator;
	3. Can use clinical prevention techniques	3. Can use clinical prevention techniques;	3. Well motivated
		4. Time less expensive than dentist	**4. Time less expensive than dentist or hygienist**
Disadvantages	**1. Time expensive**	1. Other demands on time	1. Cannot carry out clinical techniques
	2. May have poor communication skills for oral health promotion		

the planning stage and provide the basis for a switch in practice philosophy for all members of the team.

The preventive dental unit: location, function and design

In general the location for the PDU must be relaxed and friendly. Often part of a dental surgery is used as a PDU but many consider this as unwise as dental anxiety acts as a barrier to the uptake of information. Other practitioners favour waiting areas but then there is the drawback that the PDU can only be used outside of normal surgery hours. The majority of dentists agree that ideally a separate room is needed – a room specifically for the purpose of promoting oral health. It is necessary, when looking for a suitable space to locate the PDU, to consider the following questions:

1. Are there any rooms currently unused?
2. Are the uses for the rooms really necessary? For example, a large stock room would be ideal for a PDU.
3. Is there space available in existing rooms? For example partitioning off part of the waiting room for the PDU.

The function of the room should dictate its overall layout and design. The design of the PDU should be simple and reflect the type of work that will be conducted. A good example is the decision to place sinks in the PDU. This must be discussed at the outset if oral hygiene instruction is to be part of the oral health education regime. The layout and decor should facilitate a relaxed environment so that patients can listen and be encouraged to speak freely about their oral health concerns. As a wide age-range of patients will use the room it is best if the design and furnishings remain neutral. A checklist for a well-designed PDU has been developed for those dental practitioners in the planning phase.

The checklist includes:

- 'Robust fittings and furniture; work top at standard uniform height; easily cleaned work surfaces; work-top spaces for displays; easily cared for floor surfaces
- A well-lit room with a good background level for OHI, a large well-lit mirror
- Small sinks for OHI; running hot and cold water for each sink
- Good access to dental health education resources'

Oral health education resources

The type of dental health education resource will be dependent upon the philosophy underpinning oral health promotion delivery within the practice. This means that the resources should include items that allow (Table 4.7):

- the flow of information from dental health professional to patient
- the negotiation of health goals and a personalised oral health agenda for the patient

Table 4.7 Oral health promotion resources

Approach to oral health education	Necessary resources
1. Flow of oral health information	practice leaflets detailing services; practice website; leaflets and posters; other reading materials television/video presentations
2. Negotiating oral health goals	time for consultation effective communication skills
3. Teaching personal skills	effective communication skills knowledge and training in oral health promotion oral hygiene facilities; (toothbrushes, interdental cleaning agents; disclosing tablets etc.) diet history sheets motivators for children (e.g. badges, stickers) motivators for adults (e.g. oral health index)

1. Oral health information: developing reading materials

When developing information leaflets, posters or a web-site for patients, it is necessary to take into account the ease of reading, the range of facts, the layout and design of the document. Various readability indices exist which assess the ease of reading but the most common and easiest to use is the FOG [Frequency of Gobbledygook] Readability Index (Gunning 1952) (Table 4.8).

The message with leaflets and posters is to 'keep it simple'. Therefore it is best to substitute technical words with everyday words to increase understanding and readability. The fewer facts stated on the document the better, as this means that the important ones are more likely to be remembered. The simplicity of the layout and design also improves readability and recall. Blinkhorn (1993) suggests that in order to achieve this, the types of typeface, the use of italics and 'diagrams dotted about the place' should be kept to a minimum.

The development of leaflets targeting groups of patients within the practice may be beneficial. These leaflets should acknowledge the needs of the target group – for example adolescents. For example, in this patient group the emphasis should be on appearance and health-related aspects of oral health. This approach to oral health education has been shown to have positive results in the promotion of good dental health in adolescence (Redmond *et al.* 2001).

Table 4.8 How to calculate the FOG Readability Index (Blinkhorn 1993)

---

1. Randomly select samples of 100 words
2. Determine the average sentence length: number of words divided by the number of sentences
3. Determine the percentage of 'hard' words by counting the number of words of three or more syllables
4. Obtain the FOG index by adding the answers from (2) and (3) together and multiplying by 0.4
5. Add 5 to the answer to give the reading age

Example: Average sentence length = 20 words

Percentage of hard words = 10%

FOG index 0.4(10+10) = 8

Reading age 8+5 = 13 years

Increasingly, information technology is being used as a means of health education. The world-wide web and people's access to home computing mean that web-sites are increasingly being used for health promotion. Many practices have developed web-sites and use this facility as a means of promoting oral health and practice events.

2. Negotiating oral health goals

In the negotiating oral health goals, the necessary resources include effective communication skills and having time for the consultation. Concerns about having time available can act as a barrier to developing a preventive orientated practice. However there are several solutions to this apparent difficulty, such as having a dedicated member of staff who has the communication skills and the time to negotiate health goals with patients, and, the use of the 'brief intervention' technique.

The brief intervention technique has been used successfully in dental practice as part of smoking cessation programmes. The brief intervention strategy uses the 4 A's and 2 R's to shift smokers from 'pre-contemplation' to 'contemplation' and to 'preparation':

The dentist as part of a routine examination:

ASKS	the patient about their smoking habits
ADVISES	the patient to stop
ASSISTS	the patient to stop by giving leaflets about smoking cessation
ARRANGES	follow-up with the patient at the next visit and may in accordance with the patient's wishes:
REFER	the patient to a specialist service e.g. 'Quit helpline'
RECOMMEND	smoking cessation aid e.g. NRT

Evaluation of smoking cessation programmes in practice have been positive. Research suggests that up to 80 per cent of dentists rated it as a useful adjunct to their practice and were very enthusiastic about the brief intervention technique as a means of imparting oral health messages to their patients. Patients were equally enthusiastic, with over 90 per cent stating that this service should be offered by all dentists to their patients. Consequently, smoking cessation has become a recognised part of oral health promotion in practices in many practices.

3. Teaching personal oral health skills

The evidence that the teaching of oral health skills (e.g. interdental cleaning, the use of fluoride agents) can assist in promoting oral health of patients attending dental practices has been provided by Kay and Locker (1996). Dental health professionals must have expertise in the area of oral health promotion, the ability to communicate in a manner that the patient will understand and to impart information on the use of oral health hygiene products which will enable the patient to use the techniques chosen. In some instances the use of video recordings of patients have been useful in improving oral hygiene. Changes in dietary habits of children and adults have been related to the interventions tailored to the needs of the individual. The use of motivators in the guise of 'stickers' (for children) or measures of improvements in oral health status ('oral health index') for adults may help patients change their oral health regimes.

It is therefore apparent that all types of resources are needed to promote oral health in dental practice. It is not simply a case of having available information or the ability to negotiate health plans. Rather, all approaches to health education must be adopted at the chair-side.

2.3 MANAGEMENT OF THE PREVENTIVE DENTAL UNIT

It is essential that the PDU is perceived as an integral part of the dental practice. In order to foster this perception it is important that the day-to-day running of the PDU proceeds smoothly. This section will not examine the issue of choosing and ordering the resources for the PDU but restrict its focus to the areas of patient initiatives and baseline data. The gathering of baseline data on the financial implications for the practice, the effect upon patient oral health status and the views of staff is important if the performance of the PDU is to be monitored effectively. Regular practice meetings where new patient initiatives may be suggested, reports on the successes and failures of patient initiatives will allow to provide the basis for a cohesive PDU and its incorporation into the daily routines of the practice.

Baseline and final assessment information for evaluation

At the outset of the planning cycle the potential benefits of the PDU for the practice should be considered. These include a consideration of the financial benefits to the practice, the benefits to the dental team and the benefits to the patients. Furthermore, as part of the planning exercise the dentist should consider his preventive and oral health strategies to obtain his PDU goals. As part of the management of the PDU protocols must be put in place to allow the collection of baseline data (financial, patient and staff) for future evaluation of the PDU.

The financial database will consist of the expenditure on the premises, location, decoration and the equipment for the PDU. There will be daily running costs which will include staff salaries, preventive materials, oral health education resources, printing of posters and leaflets etc. An account of the financial outlay of PDU costs against the costs of routine conservation will provide a means of evaluating the effectiveness of the PDU.

The oral health status of patients must provide part of the baseline. It will be necessary to keep additional clinical records in order to assess the effects of the PDU on the promotion of oral health. This may include the use of the Oral Health Index (see Chapter 2, Section 1.8, page 87), the dmft/DMFT, and the BPE to provide baseline markers. The oral health awareness of patients with regard to their dental health knowledge must be assessed as well as their opinions for the need for a PDU. This may be done using a questionnaire and Likert-scale type questions with scores from 1 (e.g. 'I definitely don't see the point of a PDU') to 5 (e.g. 'I think it's a great idea') to assess baseline attitudes and opinions. Arrangements will need to be made to obtain further patient clinical, knowledge and attitudinal data for the evaluation of the PDU.

Staff opinions as to the success of the PDU can be gleaned during practice meetings. However, if more objective measures are required then a simple questionnaire to assess staff opinion can be administered prior to planning the PDU. Nevertheless the use of practice meetings to air concerns about the management of the PDU will have additional benefits for team building and staff cohesiveness.

Patient initiatives

The type of patient initiatives to be undertaken in the PDU will be dependent upon:
- the type and content of the oral health promotion
- the demography of the patient population
- the prevalence of oral disease
- 'Smile Week', promotional, open days for the practice

The type of oral health promotion undertaken in the practice will be dictated by the evidence-based nature of dental health education. This research-based information provides the dentist with the confidence on the success or potential failures of patient initiatives. Nevertheless whether the patient initiatives are constricted to providing knowledge (educational model) or include a health behaviour dimension (behaviour change model), the dental health education will be underpinned by the theoretical constructs associated with oral health promotion.

The demography of the patient population will affect the content of the oral health promotion. The needs of adolescent patients will be different to those of older patients with complete dentures. The awareness that patient initiatives must be tailored to the needs of the particular client again will influence the content and the type of dental health education. Although two patients may have similar oral hygiene problems their demography will dictate that the dental health education solution will be quite different. For instance the 11-year-old, who a few years earlier was so fastidious about his oral hygiene, and now rarely brushes his teeth has different needs to the 80-year-old with rheumatoid arthritis whose poor oral hygiene is related to being unable to hold a toothbrush.

The prevalence of dental disease will influence the content of patient initiatives in PDUs. Practices in poorer areas whose child patients have a high prevalence of dental caries will need to promote the use of fluoride agents and investigate dietary habits. In these situations the decision to have family oral health promotion packages in which the oral health of the child patient is seen within the wider context of the home environment may be considered. This will be in contrast to practices in higher SES areas. Nevertheless, although the patient initiatives and the dental health education materials will be of a different content and design (reflecting the differing patient and/ or practice needs) the oral health goals – to increase knowledge and/or change behaviour – will be the same.

In contrast to the routine dental health education of patients on a one-to-one basis, with patients public health campaigns such as 'Smile Week'/'No Smoking Day' or the decision to have an open day for the practice provide a different opportunity for promoting oral health. Oral health promotion within the context of the practice allows the development of promotional packages specifically tailored to the needs of the practice and provides an atmosphere for creativity and team building. Open days for the practice managed from the PDU may act as a practice builder allowing the marketing of preventive dental services.

Referral of patients, appointment times and recalls

Practice protocols agreed by the dental team for the referral of patients, together with a written prescription of care, allows for the smooth running of the PDU. As with any clinical procedure, appointment times will be allocated in accordance with the type of preventive work which is to be undertaken.

The timing of recall appointments will be influenced by the age of the patient, the prevalence of dental disease and their degree of behaviour change. The need to provide support for patients attempting to change their oral health behaviours is an important indicator of the length of time between recall appointments. Patients who are 'chronic contemplators' should be seen on a regular basis whereas patients in 'preparation' may be seen more infrequently but the length of appointment time may be longer. For those who have achieved 'maintenance' the appointments will be shorter but more intensive and participative. The timing of recall appointments will therefore not only be dependent upon the age of the patient, the prevalence of dental disease but also where the individual is on the 'stages of change model' (see fig. 4.4).

2.4 EVALUATING THE PERFORMANCE OF THE PREVENTIVE DENTAL UNIT

The final step in the planning cycle is the evaluation of the PDU. A deadline for the first evaluation of the PDU will have been set during the initial planning stage. During the evaluation stage the aims and objectives of the unit will be revisited. The baseline data from practice accounts (financial), from the practice patients' oral health status records and attitudinal data together with the views of staff members will be used and compared with data collected for the purpose of evaluation.

At the outset of the evaluation the aim of the PDU must be assessed. This may be done by re-examining the goal setting which formed part of the planning stage – has the practice orientation changed from being a restoratively to preventatively orientated practice? What are the aims for the future? (fig. 4.5).

In order to assess how far the practice has come in terms of achieving its goals the evaluation must also assess the benefits of the PDU for the practice in terms of:

1. Has the PDU benefited the financial standing of the practice?

This aspect of the evaluation has been described as 'financial housekeeping'. As a result of keeping an effective book-keeping and accounting system it will be possible to monitor the annual costs of the PDU. However, a distinction must be made with regard to the short-term compared with long term financial goals. In the short-term consideration will have to be made for the capital expenditure (building costs, equipment costs, decoration costs, staff costs) and the costs for oral health materials and resources. These costs will be off-set against the savings in terms of patient treatment costs, the revenue

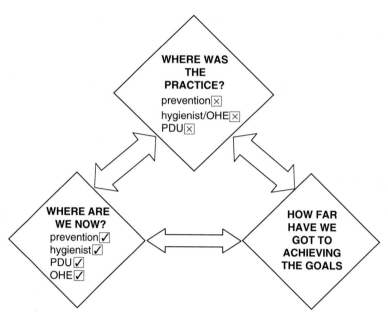

Figure 4.5 Evaluating and setting future goals for the PDU.

from attracting new patients and selling more oral health products. In the short-term the financial goals may be to reduce the costs on the loan for the PDU. However to achieve the long term goal of a financially viable PDU, the recurrent costs of the unit must become integrated into the practice's annual business plan so that the goal of profitability may be obtained.

2. Has the PDU benefited the patients?

The means of assessing this benefit is clear cut. It involves examining changes in their oral health knowledge, attitudes and oral health status. Issues raised by patients – for example the times of opening of the PDU or the appropriateness of the oral health education aids – will allow the unit to be fine-tuned and to be responsive to the needs of the community it serves.

3. Has the PDU benefited the practice staff?

The benefits for the staff may be continuously re-evaluated. These will include increase in job satisfaction and a decrease in occupational stress. Regular staff meetings provide the forum for discussions on the pros and cons of the PDU as well as the airing of new strategies and ideas to be incorporated into the preventive practice. At these meetings an opportunity is presented to discuss the further evaluation of the PDU and how it can retain its evolving character.

The evaluation of the PDU represents an important part of the life of the dental practice. Failures in reaching health goals are as important as reasons of attainment. Both must be incorporated into the action plan and used as a basis for future planning and development of the PDU. Assessing dental practice in this way allows the sustained development of the preventive orientated practice within an ever-evolving dental health care situation.

2.5 CONCLUSIONS

The aim of this section was to present theories of health promotion, health education and health behaviours as a means of providing practice policy to allow the development of an integrated approach to promoting oral health in general dental practice. Using oral health promotion theory as a backdrop it suggested that in order to develop an effective PDU the opinions and attitudes of the stakeholders in terms of the benefits to the practice, the patients and staff had to be considered. The PDU would therefore cater for the needs of the patient community it served while providing an arena for practice building and staff cohesion. The need to evaluate regularly the effectiveness of the PDU could be considered as being central to the sustained development of an integrated oral health dental practice.

3.0 USE OF MINIMALLY INVASIVE TECHNIQUES (MI)

Minimal or non-intervention techniques are in general preferred by patients as they tend to be quicker and painless. Practice building means telling patients about minimal intervention, and, in the case of non-intervention, or a 'wait and see' approach, that the patient has responsibilities such as the consumption of a non-cariogenic diet and the maintenance of good plaque control.

Minimal intervention techniques include, Atraumatic Restorative Treatment (ART), the Preventive Resin Restoration (PRR), the Class II resin-composite in the initial cavity as opposed to the Black's Class II amalgam cavity and the dentine-bonded crown. However, before a decision to intervene is made, the clinician should be certain that intervention is indicated.

3.1 TREATMENT OF THE INITIAL CARIES LESION

Correct diagnosis and treatment of carious lesions is central to clinical dental practice. Accordingly, a dental practitioner may spend much of his/her

surgery time either,
- deciding whether lesions of caries are present,
- accumulating information for each particular patient in order to make a judgement on how to treat such lesions, or,
- if restoration of the caries is indicated, how the caries should be restored.

The clinicians' dilemma is therefore **prevention** versus **restoration.**

Given that approximately 70% of restorations are replacements of existing restorations, the importance of the decision of whether to treat an initial carious lesion is of paramount importance, given that the cutting of tooth substance and its ultimate restoration commits the tooth to a lifetime programme of restorative treatment. There are a series of decisions that the clinician must make, prior to committing the tooth to a restoration.

The carious process commences as subsurface demineralisation which, following periods of remineralisation and demineralisation, may progress or arrest.

First, the clinician must make a diagnosis – is a caries lesion present? There are several factors of relevance to this:
- the tooth surface should be clean and dry for easy recognition of the initial lesion
- on a smooth surface the initial lesion appears as a 'white spot'
- older caries lesions take up stains and become brown
- fibre optic transillumination and bitewing radiographs may help diagnose proximal caries
- tooth separation techniques may be useful, but require two visits approximately one week apart.
- newer methods of caries detection include electronic caries detectors and variable frequency AC impedance spectroscopy
- radiographic evidence of caries will underestimate the extent of the histological lesion.

Second, the clinician must decide – is the caries active or not? There are several further questions of relevance to this:
- is the caries through enamel into dentine?
- what distance has it travelled into dentine?
- is the lesion cavitated?

As a general rule, if the extent of caries is accurately diagnosed, for non-cavitated lesions in enamel and extending up to one-third of the dentine width, an attempt should be made at remineralisation, providing that this can be justified in the light of the patient's caries risk status. While accurate diagnosis is fundamental, the calculation of the patient's caries risk status is the second most important consideration when caries has been diagnosed.

Important factors in risk assessment for caries (RAC) are shown in Table 4.9.

Risk assessment for caries has been considered to be a developing science because most risk factors, individually, have low predictive value. However, it could be anticipated from Table 4.9 that a patient who has low fluoride

Table 4.9 Important factors in risk assessment for caries (RAC)

Factor:	fluoride availability at the time and site of demineralisation
Relevance:	fluoride availability has been considered to be more important than systemic uptake during tooth formation.
Factor:	dietary sucrose intake
Relevance:	A cariogenic diet has not yet been defined, but sugar intake and frequency of snacking have both been strongly related to caries activity.
Factor:	likely patient compliance with dietary advice
Relevance:	Patient compliance with dietary advice may be difficult to determine given that human nature will make under recording of sugar intake the norm; the response to oral hygiene instruction is more readily visualised. Readiness to change behaviour should also be considered.
Factor:	the presence of caries lesions and restorations
Relevance:	It has been considered that the best identifiable risk factor is the presence of an active caries lesion (Suddick and Dodds 1997), while in the San Antonio CRA procedure, caries and fillings are both viewed as predictors of risk, but lesions are weighted more highly than fillings.
Factor:	adequacy of salivary flow
Relevance:	Salivary flow measurements may be carried out for those patients for whom reduced salivary flow is suspected. Reduced salivary flow may be considered to predispose to caries, especially in patients who have not complied with dietary advice.
Factor:	dental attendance patterns
Relevance:	Dental attendance patterns are not so much a predictor of caries risk, but of the risk of further development of the untreated lesion, given that the poor attender is less likely to attend for either preventive or restorative treatment.
Factor:	result of *mutans streptococci* tests
Relevance:	*Mutans streptococci* (MS) are among the organisms causing primary caries lesions. A negative salivary MS test indicates lack of caries activity while a positive MS test may indicate a caries active patient.

availability at the time and site of demineralisation, high dietary sucrose intake, poor compliance with dietary and oral hygiene advice, who has reduced salivary flow, is an irregular dental attender, has a high *mutans streptococci* (MS) count and who already has active caries, would be at high risk for further caries. Reducing the number of risk factors may reduce the risk, but the influence of each factor may vary with each patient.

It has been considered that the following factors contribute to increasing risk of developing new caries lesions (Suddick and Dodds 1997):

- prior caries incidence
- frequent intake of sugary foods or snacks
- not living in fluoridated community and not using fluoride dentrifice
- age (i.e. child, adolescent)
- low unstimulated salivary flow
- high salivary MS count

This information should be, with the possible exception of the quantitative assessment of MS, available to the dental practitioner in his/her dental office. It should therefore be possible to identify the at-risk patient with reasonable accuracy, and consequently, to make a decision on the need – or otherwise – to restore a caries lesion. The decision *not* to restore should signal the commencement of preventive therapy, ultimately followed by the assessment of whether a particular lesion is active or not at a time determined by the RAC. The decision to restore is followed by the choice of the most appropriate restorative material.

3.2   MINIMAL INTERVENTION (MI) TECHNIQUES

Minimal intervention in the treatment of children

The management of caries in the primary dentition is an important aspect of general practice dentistry, and this may take the form of making cavities self-cleansing in the hope that the caries will arrest if the diet can be made non-cariogenic, or it may take the form of supervised non-treatment. Leaving caries untreated is never appropriate, but the level of emotional maturity, previous dental experience and the influence of the family, the dental surgery environment and the dental team all affect how an individual child with dental caries is managed.

Stabilisation using minimal tooth tissue removal can be used as part of a holistic approach to the management of a pre-cooperative or anxious child. Dressing the tooth with a fluoride leaching material may buy time by slowing the progress of disease whilst the child learns how to cope with dental treatment. Then the general dental practitioner has two basic choices:

- to carry our excavation of caries and restore the defect with a fluoride-containing material, adopting the Atraumatic Restorative Treatment (ART) approach
- administer local anaesthesia and restore the cavity with a classical Black's style Class I or II restoration in amalgam, or, a stainless steel crown.

It could be expected that there would be benefits in respect of patient (and parent) co-operation when the ART approach is employed and it could also be expected that in general the child patient will be less anxious when the clinician adopts the ART approach.

The ART technique was pioneered in the mid-1980s in Tanzania and further developed in a community field trial in Thailand in 1991 and in another community field trial in Zimbabwe in 1993. The technique has been described by Frencken and co-workers in a World Health Organisation booklet (1997), who state that the two main principles of ART are:

- Removing carious tooth tissues using only hand instruments, such as spoon excavators, and
- Restoring the cavity with a material that adheres to the tooth.

The original concept was that the technique allowed dentistry to be carried out in less industrialised areas of countries where the supply of electricity may be unreliable, but there would seem to be no reason why it could not be adopted in general dental practices worldwide.

Currently glass-ionomer is the restorative material with which ART is performed (Mjor and Gordan 1999). The reasons for using hand instruments rather than electric handpieces are that it makes restorative care accessible to all population groups, it conserves tooth tissue and reduces the need for local anaesthesia to a minimum. Additionally, infection control is simplified as hand instruments can readily be cleaned and sterilised and, the cost of hand instruments is low, compared with handpieces.

Results of a recent survey of UK dentists indicated that, although almost half of the respondents stated that they were aware of the ART technique, few were applying the ART technique in its true form (i.e. removal of caries without a drill and without a need for LA) in their clinical practice, with hand excavation alone being proposed by less than 10% of the respondents to the survey and approximately half suggesting the use of a drill and 40% using an excavator and drill in combination. However, over half of the respondents did use materials which are associated with an adhesive approach, namely glass-ionomer and compomer (Burke *et al.* 2002).

Reasons for the less than complete adoption of the ART minimal intervention approach may be:

- That UK dentists considered that ART is only appropriate to the areas for which it was originally considered suitable, namely in un-industrialised countries, rather than in practices in the UK.
- They may also have considered that use of a drill was faster than ART.

MI in the treatment of adolescents and adults

It could be considered that minimal preparation techniques should be employed for treatment of adults and adolescents, as well as children. However, as no treatment is arguably the least intervention, correct diagnosis in respect of when and whether intervention is indicated is central to the concept of MI. For correct diagnosis of fissure caries, the following are of relevance:

- Visual inspection, with well lit (possibly by fibre-optic), clean, dry field and magnification
- Use of a sharp probe is neither reliable or appropriate
- Radiography may provide diagnostic confirmation in detection and progress

Methods available for caries diagnosis are shown in Table 4.10, but none has achieved widespread acceptance other than visual examination.

The patients' caries risk is related to their present and past history of the disease. However, when caries is diagnosed, the risk of development of further lesions and increase in size of existing lesions is related to:

- Caries history
- Current fluoride status
- Current dietary status
- Saliva and microbiological considerations
- Current behaviour in respect of patient attendance and cooperation

When a decision has been made to intervene, based on RAC (risk assessment for caries) (Table 4.9), minimal preparation techniques should be employed wherever possible. Adhesive materials and techniques have improved the capability of the restorative dentist to treat the initial caries lesion in a conservative manner. The lack of bonding capability of amalgam makes it unsuitable for the restoration of the minimal caries lesion, given that the achievement of adequate resistance and retention form for such an amalgam restoration may require removal of considerable amounts of sound tooth substance. The use of materials which may be bonded to tooth substance is therefore indicated for the treatment of initial caries. MI cavity designs such as the Preventive Resin Restoration (PRR) show high potential for success. The use of magnification during the preparation for the PRR is highly recommended. Additionally, it could be considered that resin composite, using an adhesive cavity design is the material of choice for the initial class II caries lesion, because of the substantial amounts of tooth substance that may be saved when a minimal cavity design is employed (fig. 4.6).

Table 4.10 Methods for caries diagnosis

Visual inspection
Radiography
Electrical resistance (ECM)
Quantitative Laser and Light Fluorescence (QLF)
Infra Red Laser Fluorescence
Light transmission (FOTI)

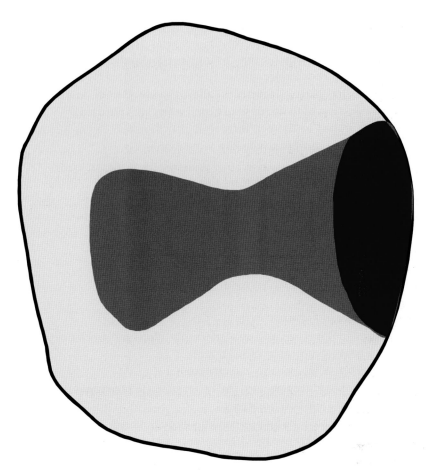

Figure 4.6 Tooth substance saved (dark blue) when a MI cavity design for resin composite is employed, as compared with a conventional class II design. (Reproduced by courtesy of George Warman Publications, Guildford, Surrey, UK, publishers of Dental Update.)

Air abrasion

Air abrasion is an alternative method for minimal preparation of caries cavities. Current devices use a stream of Al_2O_3 particles generated from compressed air or bottled CO_2 or N_2. Efficiency of cutting is related to hardness of tissue, with pressures of 40–160 pounds/sq.inch being used. It is also dependent on the speed of particles when they hit the tooth and this is related to gas pressure, nozzle diameter, particle size and distance from tooth.

Uses of air abrasion include
- Removal of superficial enamel defects
- Preparation of fissures for sealants
- Preparation for PRR

- Surface preparation of Class V
- Removal of fissure surface stains
- Cleaning of tooth structure and castings for cementation or bonding
- Detection of pit and fissure caries

Air abrasion has been considered to allow visualisation of, and access to, caries with less loss of tooth substance than when burs are used.

If caries limited to enamel, then sealant or flowable composite may be placed, if dentine is involved then PRR is appropriate.

Advantages of air abrasion include

- A high proportion of patients do not require LA
- Discomfort may be managed by reducing air pressure and powder flow
- Patients are less anxious with the sound of air abrasion, compared to turbine
- There is no vibration
- Air abrasion may remove less tooth substance than drill

Disadvantages of air abrasion include:

- It is not suited for removal of amalgam restorations and gross caries
- There is a risk of laceration of soft tissues
- There is a risk of air embolus via soft tissues
- Air abrasion produces rounded cavity not suited to preparations requiring definitive walls and sharp margins
- It does not obviate need for acid conditioning of enamel
- The clinician and his/her staff need to learn a new clinical technique
- The cost of purchasing an air abrasion machine, although some are now available for less than £1000
- The abrasive dust may gather on surgery surfaces

Nevertheless, despite these disadvantages, increasing numbers of dentists are adding this method of tooth preparation to their armamentarium.

Chemomechanical methods of tooth preparation

Chemical means of caries removal, such as Carisolv (Medi Team, S-433 63, Savedalen, Sweden), may be appropriate to minimal intervention, and is patient-friendly, as local anaesthesia is rarely indicated. Carisolv employs a variety of amino acids in a solution of sodium hypochlorite (Table 4.11).

The clinical technique for Carisolv involves administration of local anaesthesia only if patient requests it, removal of overlying enamel, if required, with rotary instruments, application of Carisolv to carious dentine, waiting for 30 seconds and the use of specially designed double-sided excavators scrape the caries away. The area is then cleaned to inspect for caries removal, and the procedure repeated as required. Advantages include excellent patient acceptance and the need to use LA only occasionally, while disadvantages

Table 4.11 Constituents of Carisolv (Medi Team, S-433 63, Savedalen, Sweden)

Clear liquid	*Red gel (pH 11)*
NaOCl	3 amino acids:
	Leucine
	Lycine
	Glutamic acid
	Carboxymethyl-cellulose gel
	Na (OH)$_2$
	Colouring agent

include the lengthier treatment time as compared with cavity preparation with rotary instruments and the cost of the solution.

MI with dentine-bonded crowns

A dentine-bonded crown may be defined as a full coverage restoration in which an all-ceramic crown is bonded to the underlying dentine (and any available enamel) using a resin composite luting material, with the bond being mediated by the use of a dentine-bonding system and a micromechanically retentive ceramic fitting surface. There are therefore a number of components to this technique, namely (Burke *et al.* 1998) (fig. 4.7):

- The use of a ceramic for the construction of the crown which allows etching with HF to create a micromechanically retentive fit surface to the crown: these include feldspathic porcelain, aluminous porcelain and Empress (Ivoclar Vivadent: Liechtenstein)
- The treatment of the etched ceramic fit surface with a silane coupling agent to improve the bond between the ceramic and the resin luting material
- The treatment of the dentine surface of the prepared tooth with a minimal film thickness dentine bonding agent
- The use of a dual-cure resin luting material

Dentine-bonded crowns use similar technology to that employed in the construction and fitting of porcelain veneers. Indeed, the technique could be considered to be a veneer on the labial and on the palatal aspect of the prepared tooth. Preparation is therefore minimal, with a crown thickness as low as 1 mm being appropriate. It could therefore be considered that the dentine-bonded crown technique uses the dentine as the core, as opposed to alumina (in the aluminous porcelain crown), metal (in the porcelain-fused-to-metal crown) or leucite (in the Empress crown). Advantages include the need for only minimal tooth preparation, the potential for good aesthetics

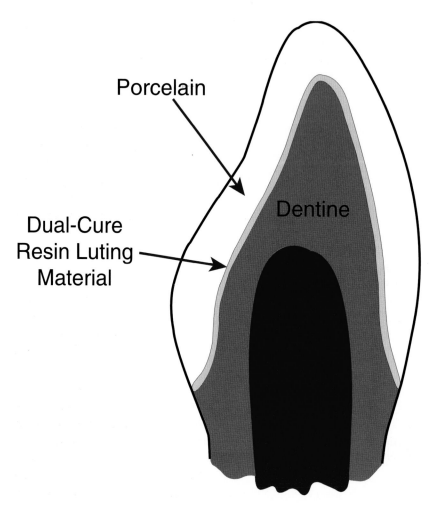

Figure 4.7 The components of a dentine-bonded crown (reproduced by courtesy of George Warman Publications, Guildford, Surrey, UK, publishers of Dental Update). White-feldspathic porcelain, with fitting surface made micromechanically retentive by etching with HF. Blue line – dual cure resin luting cement. Light blue – dentine treated by dentine bonding agent. Dark blue – pulp.

(because there is no metal core), good fracture resistance, the reliable means by which the crown is bonded to the tooth and the low solubility of the resin luting material. Disadvantages include the need to carry out occlusal adjustment after placement (because adjustment of these thin ceramic crowns extra-orally could lead to ceramic fracture), and the more technique sensitive nature of the crown placement, as compared with cementation with conventional cements, because of the need to etch and then bond with a dentine-bonding agent during placement. However, the employment of new self-adhesive resin cements (such as Unicem:3M ESPE, Seefeld, Germany) which do not require etching and bonding to gain adhesion to the dentine surface, should reduce technique sensitivity during placement of dentine-bonded crowns.

Long term provisional restorations

Glass ionomer and compomer materials may have indications for patients who request a tooth-coloured restoration which are prepared to accept a long term provisional restoration which may be placed at reduced cost as compared to other tooth-coloured restorations such as direct-placement resin-composite, for nervous, phobic patients in whom the use of materials which may be more time-consuming or technique sensitive to place may be precluded.

Summary

In summary, the treatment of the initial lesion of caries, albeit an everyday occurrence for the dental practitioner, presents considerable demands of patient assessment and diagnosis. Whatever decisions are made – to restore the caries or to attempt to arrest its progress – the adoption of a maintenance programme is of paramount importance. Patient motivation, in respect of dietary control and satisfactory oral hygiene, is central to a successful outcome, and, in future, practice management programmes may include RAC as a diagnostic aid. New methods of management of caries lesions are more dynamic than traditional methods and place restoration of the lesion towards the bottom of the list of possible treatments, with the biologic rather than the mechanistic approach being a priority. However, changes in the teaching of RAC in dental schools and in the third-party funding of diagnostic tests and diagnosis also requires re-appraisal in order to reflect the increasing complexity of management of the initial caries lesion. If restorative intervention is indicated following diagnosis and RAC, treatment of the caries should be by a minimal-intervention adhesive technique.

4.0 CARING FOR PATIENTS WITH SPECIAL DENTAL NEEDS IN PRIMARY CARE

The term 'special need' has come to represent individuals who experience difficulties in their lives. People described by this term are a disparate group since their special need may be a result of chronic physical or mental illness; physical disability; learning difficulties; injecting drug use; dental phobia or sensory impairment. Individuals who are described by the various categories of special need do not represent a homogenous group – for instance some may have lesser or greater degrees of disability or impairment. The consequence of perceiving people with special needs as a homogenous group has provided the basis for incorrect views, opinions and prejudices to those described as 'handicapped'. The reduced and restricted access to primary care can be seen within a framework of social exclusion (Freeman, 2002).

It is in the nature of social exclusion that those who are excluded also have the worst health. They have greater experience of ill health, work-related illnesses and accidents, a higher prevalence of alcoholism, injecting drug use and premature morbidity. When these health facts are coupled with the restricted access to primary care it seems that those with the greatest [health] need are in receipt of inappropriate health services. Therefore there is the potential for what is known as an 'inverse care law' to exist for this client group. This corpus of special need with social exclusion and reduced access to primary care has particular relevance for dental health. The need for dentists in general practice to provide accessible dental health care for people with special needs in their practice populations is an urgent consideration. In order that this goal may be achieved it is necessary to consider a strategy based upon a model of accessibility in which access to dental care is perceived as a balance between enabling and inhibiting factors. Cohen (1987) in her review of the FDI's classification of access to dental care described a three-level model composed of 'accessibility factors'. The model viewed access to primary care in relation to the society, the health professional and patient. Access to primary dental care could, therefore, be described in terms of psycho-social need, work demands and societal concerns (Table 4.12).

It would seem appropriate that, in order to increase accessibility, government and health professionals groups should have an awareness of the need for responsive primary care services. Doing so will allow the FDI's

---

Table 4.12 FDI's classification of accessibility factors

Accessibility factors	
1. Society and government factors	Insufficient public support of attitudes conducive to health, inadequate oral health care facilities, inadequate oral health manpower and insufficient support for research'
2. Dental profession factors	'Inappropriate manpower resources, uneven geographical distribution, training inappropriate to changing needs and demands and insufficient sensitivity to patient's attitudes and needs'
3. Patient factors	'Lack of perceived need, anxiety and fear, financial considerations and lack of access'

accessibility model to be converted from policy to strategy to implementation in the primary care sector. However to achieve this goal would mean that the government and society would need to provide an environment in which accessing dental services was easy for those with special needs. This could only be achieved by government putting in place legislation to reduce discrimination, ensuring equitable distribution of oral health services, adequate oral health care facilities and adequate oral health manpower. This is starting to happen. Secondly, within this 'healthier environment', there would be a need for appropriately trained dental personnel to connect with people's special needs and to be sensitive to their fears and concerns (dental professional factors) and thirdly, to relate to the individual patient's difficulties with being able to access and accept primary dental care.

The aim of this section is to examine each of the above accessibility factors with regard to the provision of primary dental care for those with special needs. Factors relating to the patient in terms of perceived need, anxiety and fear, financial considerations and lack of access have been considered elsewhere (Chapters 1 and 2). This section will examine aspects of government legislation (e.g. the Disability Discrimination Act), accessibility factors related to the practice (e.g. the physical layout and dimensions of the practice) and their personnel (e.g. attitudes of the dental team) and, finally, clinical decision making with respect to providing appropriate dental care for special needs patients in the primary care setting.

4.1 SOCIETY AND GOVERNMENT FACTORS

Disability has popularly been viewed as an illness which was described in terms of the medical model. Disability within the medical model framework was perceived as a 'something' for which a bio-medical solution could be found. However, the social model of disability suggests that society rather than impairment disables people. Society does this by excluding disabled people from their rights of employment, education and access to goods, facilities and services and as society oppresses those with disability then society must change if the stigma of disability is to be ameliorated. The Government has recently introduced the report 'NHS dentistry: options for change' (DH 2002) and the Disability Discrimination Act (DfES 1995). While the Act views disability within the social model and promotes social change as a means of reducing social exclusion and access to goods, facilities and services, 'Options for change' stresses the importance of access to dental care as mainstream in reducing oral health inequalities. It would seem therefore that the 'Options for change' report (DH 2002) and the Disability Discrimination Act (DfES 1995) will have important ramifications for those in primary dental care (Merry and Edwards 2002).

Government legislation: NHS dentistry: options for change (DH 2002)

The publication of the government document – 'NHS dentistry: options for change' has allowed the theme of providing accessible dental care for those with special needs to take centre stage. The report aims to modernise dentistry by allowing *'the dental team to focus on preventive measures to combat dental disease, and to tackle serious oral health inequalities'*. The report stresses the need to change methods of remuneration, improve dental education and provide clinical pathways underpinned by clinical governance in order to provide access and evidence-based primary health care for all who wish it. 'Options for change' (DH 2002) particularly emphasises the need to find care options to maintain the oral health of those with special needs by using patient-focused strategies. These strategies are not perceived as forming part of a safety-net service, but are viewed as mainstream in the wish to reduce oral health inequality. Increasing accessibility and the focus on those with special needs is apparent. 'NHS dentistry: Options for Change' (DH 2002) states that:

> 'access will be secured for those . . . with special needs, wanting
> - regular dental care with a dentist of their choice
> - dental care when having trouble (including out of hours and care needed urgently)
> - specialist care'

Government legislation: the Disability Discrimination Act (DfES 1995)

In 1995 the Government introduced a series of new laws to reduce discrimination and to give new rights of access to goods, facilities and services. Intrinsic to the Act is the acknowledgement that people with special needs must have the same employment, education and access to goods, facilities, services and premises as those without disability. Essentially the Act is divided into 3 parts. The first part provides a comprehensive definition of disability (introduced January 1996), the second part deals with employment legislation (introduced October 1999) and the third part examines access to goods, facilities, services and premises (to be introduced in 2004).

Definitions of Disability

The Act's defines disability as a person with *'a physical or mental impairment which has a substantial and long term adverse effect on his ability to carry out normal day-to-day activities'*. The Act's definition of disability is similar to that of the World Health Organisation (WHO) (Barbotte *et al.* 2001) which defines disability as '*A restriction or inability to perform an activity in the manner or within the range considered normal for a human being, mostly resulting from impairment*'. The Act does not furnish the reader with a definition of impairment but a useful definition is provided by the WHO (Barbotte *et al.* 2001). They state that impairment is, '*Any temporary or permanent loss or abnormality of a body structure or function, whether physiological or psychological. An impairment is a disturbance affecting functions that are essentially mental or sensory, internal organs, the head, the trunk or the limbs*'.

Within the Act's definition of disability are those who have a learning disability, mental illness, sensory impairment, physical illness and physical disability. The Act acknowledges that those with impaired liver functioning due to chronic alcoholism have a disability but it is due to liver disease and not the alcoholism. Therefore it is interesting to note that the Act's definition excludes those who are, for example, alcoholics, injecting drug users but who are nevertheless included in the wider definition of special need.

Elimination of discrimination in the field of employment

The purpose of this part of the Act is to protect disabled people from discrimination and that employers must '*make reasonable adjustments if their employment arrangements or premises place disabled people at substantial disadvantage compared with non-disabled people*'.

Discrimination during employment can occur as a result of an employer:

a) providing different terms of employment (e.g. salary) for the disabled compared with the non-disabled employee
b) in differing career opportunities (e.g. promotion) for the disabled compared with the non-disabled employee
c) refusing or deliberately avoiding affording the disabled employee of career opportunities
d) dismissing or subjecting the disabled employee to derision or detriment.
   Discrimination in employment can therefore occur in one of two ways:
- first by the employer treating the disabled person less favourably than the non-disabled employee, and
- secondly by failing to comply with a period of induction and making adjustments (e.g. working hours) for the disabled employee.

In order to reduce the likelihood of discrimination the Act advises employers (e.g. dentists) to be flexible, consult with the disabled person, seek expert opinion, plan ahead and promote equal opportunities.

Rights of access to goods, facilities, services, and premises

The third part of the Act becomes law in 2004. This part of the Act states clearly that disabled people must have rights of access to goods, facilities, services and premises as non-disabled people. In many ways this part of the Act mirrors the second part. Service providers, like employers, will have to make reasonable adjustments to their premises to reduce physical barriers to increase accessibility for the disabled individual.

Discrimination may occur when the disabled person is treated in a less favourable way because of her disability compared with others. This may occur by refusing to treat the individual, providing a lower standard of care and/or on worse terms. In addition, if physical adjustments are not made to premises to accommodate, for example, wheelchairs, then because of the lack of physical access the disabled person is being discriminated against. Acknowledging the need for clear practice policies and procedures as well as the provision of alternative means of making available services for disabled people will promote equal opportunity. Discussions with disabled clients and experts in the area of special needs will also provide an environment in which the disabled individual will not feel discriminated against.

Implications for primary dental care

In the United Kingdom 6.8 million adults are considered to have a disability. The need to provide appropriate employment opportunities and health facilities for those who are disabled has become an important policy issue. Within the rubric of the Primary Health Care Approach (WHO 1978) the requirement for health care facilities to be accessible, available, acceptable, affordable and appropriate has allowed an examination of oral health care facilities for patients and employees with special needs.

The employment legislation has already been commented upon (see: Elimination of discrimination in the field of employment), however this part of the Act has implications for dentists employing staff. Dentists must be knowledgeable and comply with the employment legislation of the Act.

With regard to the provision of primary dental care there is little doubt that the majority of dental practitioners believe that it is appropriate and within their clinical remit to care for and to treat patients with special needs. However, various surveys of general dental practices have shown that the surgery premises lack the physical amenities to enable easy access. Outside the surgery building, the majority of practices do not have wheelchair access, ramps or lifts to surgery entrances while inside; it is only a minority that has accessible cloakrooms, lavatories and waiting rooms (Freeman *et al.* 1997, Edwards and Merry 2002). Despite attempts to improve accessibility by providing domiciliary care many practitioners felt poorly trained and equipped to treat patients in their own homes (Edwards and Merry 2002). It seemed that dentists were unable to take full advantage of this alternative and appropriate strategy to increase accessibility for this patient population. The available evidence would suggest that the lack of access to primary dental care services and premises contravenes the third part of the Disability Discrimination Act (DfES 1995).

Merry and Edwards (2002) give an excellent commentary on the Act and highlight the policies, procedures and physical adjustments which must be made so that dentists in primary dental care can comply with part 3 of the Act. They in particular point out the need for dentists to be aware of providing reasonable adjustments to their practices. This may include reducing physical barriers to their surgery (e.g. installing a ramp) premises as well as providing '*large print leaflets for the partially sighted patient*' and/or '*one member of to have some [sensory impairment] equality training*'.

The Disability Rights Commission has provided a checklist of good practice (Table 4.13) to ensure compliance with the Act and when checklist is combined with Merry and Edwards' (2002) commentary on the Act they provide the dentist in primary care with the means of complying with the Disability Discrimination Act (DfES 1995).

4.2 DENTAL HEALTH PROFESSIONAL FACTORS

The role of the dental health professional as part of the primary health care team has been implicated as pertinent in providing an accessible service for

Table 4.13 Check-list of good practice (DfES 1995)

1. 'Think and plan ahead to meet the requirements of your disabled patients.
2. Don't make assumptions about disabled people based in speculation or stereotypes. Think about the wide range of disabilities that there are when planning adjustments.
3. If in doubt, ask disabled people themselves how they can best be served. Listen carefully and respond to what they really want. You could consult with disabled staff and disability organisations.
4. Think about the way you treat disabled patients. Let them know how to request for assistance.
5. Ensure that you respect the dignity of a disabled person when providing them with services.
6. Establish a practice policy on providing services to ensure it includes providing appropriate care for disabled people. Communicate and discuss this policy with the dental team and staff members.
7. Make sure that your staff is knowledgeable about the Act and disabled people's legal rights. Ensure that the dental team has taken part in disability awareness and disability etiquette training.
8. Regularly review your surgery premises and policies to maintain high accessibility for disabled patients'.

those with special needs. The requirement for primary dental care services to merge with primary health care services has been seen as essential to the provision of health care for all. Central to this is the view that it is the culture of dental practice with its system of payment, the poverty of positive attitudes and inadequate dental education which contribute to the lack of accessible primary dental care in the general practice setting.

Methods of financial remuneration

Describing methods of payment, Oliver and Nunn (1996) show that 'fee-per-item' acts as a financial disincentive to accepting physically disabled people as general practice patients. They have pointed to the dilemma stating that this is a direct result of the current method of remuneration and postulates the need for discretionary fees for practitioners if adults with special needs are to access appropriate dental health care services. The need for dentists in primary care, therefore, to be provided with additional and alternative payment systems has been considered central to reducing barriers to care for those with special needs. The Government (DH 2002) has now acknowledged that:

> 'Patient charges are a driver of health inequalities [*and*] those in the greatest need are least likely to access the service and often pay the most for their dental care'

Alternative payment systems have been recognised by the DH (2002) and include sessional payments, capitation, dental payment cards, fee-per-item or a combination of these; the integration of salaried and fee-per-item services into primary dental care services and the separation of patient charges from dentists' fees and the collection of charges. It has been proposed that these changes in remuneration would assist in reducing the barrier of costs of dental treatment to provide responsive dental care for those with special needs.

Attitudes of dental health professionals

The attitudes of dental health professionals to those with special needs have been highlighted as a factor in reducing access to care. At the centre of the concerns felt by general practitioners are fears of reduced income due to reduced through-put of patients, increased turnaround time and patients going elsewhere for treatment. Concerns for the welfare of the practice together with anxieties about their own health have been shown to be predictive in providing care for HIV-seropositive patients (Gibson and Freeman 1996a). Nevertheless, although dentists experienced such concerns and worries in areas of high prevalence of HIV their negative attitudes were over-ridden by the wish to provide care for this patient population (Gibson and Freeman 1996b). Hence despite having negative attitudes these general dental practitioners provided dental treatment for HIV seropositive patients who attended their surgeries.

Postgraduate training

The scarcity of high-street specialists in special needs dentistry has been illustrated by Olivier and Nunn (1996) and highlights the requirement for undergraduate and postgraduate dental education. While it is not necessary to describe the elements of undergraduate training it is important to note that graduates' decision to treat special needs patients in practice was associated with increased confidence and their ability to care for the disabled during their undergraduate clinical experience. Furthermore, with regard to providing domiciliary care services, lack of adequate training, confidence and concerns about equipment were identified as barriers to the provision of domiciliary care by those in primary dental care (Edwards and Merry 2002). The British Society for Disability and Oral Health guidelines and recommendations for domiciliary dental care services (Fiske and Lewis 2000) have insisted on the need for 'teamwork'. These have emphasised the importance of specialised knowledge and skills for each member of the dental team. The necessary skills ranged from map reading and navigation to flexibility, improvisation, manual handling and basic life support. The recommendation that all dental team members have training to develop and maintain their confidence and ability in the provision of domiciliary dental care is stated in the British Society for Disability and Oral Health guidelines (Fiske and Lewis 2000).

The Royal College of Surgeons (2001) has supported the call for an integrated approach for those with learning difficulties. They extrapolate this need and demand that those involved in every aspect of dental treatment, including professions complimentary to dentistry and other health care professionals must have specialist training. The Certificate in Special Care Dental Nursing is illustrative and provides dental nurses with specialist training in the care of special needs patients.

The acquisition of skills, the ability and confidence to treat must be central to any postgraduate training in this subject area. Special needs dentistry is considered an essential part of continuing professional development (Royal College of Surgeons 2001). There is a need for formal and informal courses with elements of self-directed learning for dentists, and this is indicated to increase awareness, improve attitudes, confidence and access to care.

Inequitable distribution of services: domiciliary dental care services

Inequitable distribution of services is usually thought of in terms of geographic location with people accessing health clinics which are in a 5-kilometre radius of their place of residence. However there are patient populations (Table 4.14) who, because of physical disabilities and/or mental impairment, find it extremely difficult or impossible to attend for dental surgery-based care.

Table 4.14 Patient groups possibly requiring domiciliary dental care services (Fiske and Lewis 2000)

- Physical disabilities causing problems with motility
- Medical conditions leading to disability: chronic obstructive airways disease, emphysema, stroke, Parkinson's disease
- Conditions that make them disorientated, confused or panicked when removed from familiar environment – such as autism, Alzheimer's disease, agoraphobia
- Learning difficulties or mental disability that causes difficulty in making and keeping appointment times
- Severe dental anxiety or phobia that people feel unable to enter a dental surgery

Groups of patients such as those residing in long stay accommodation or being cared for by relatives in their own homes, for example, may need to rely on alternative forms of primary dental services. Fiske and Lewis (2000) have stated that, as people live longer, the requirement for domiciliary care will increase. Furthermore, the urgency to provide appropriate primary care has increased as it has been shown that this patient population has greater experience of ill-health and unmet treatment need as a consequence of being unable to access primary surgery-based dental services.

Domiciliary dental care services have been considered as a means of providing primary dental care for housebound patients. Burke *et al.* (1995) assessed the availability of domiciliary dental services provided by general dental practitioners. Their results indicated that the vast majority of dentists provided domiciliary dental care outside the usual working day. It seems that on average a primary care dentist will provide domiciliary dental care for nearly 3 patients per month. In general, the categories of treatment provided tend to include oral hygiene procedures, dentures, extractions and simple restorations.

Furthermore, dentists who have previously provided domiciliary care not only intended to do so in the future but perceived domiciliary dental care as a valuable asset to their general practice. It seemed (as mentioned previously) that the need for adequate remuneration, continuing professional development and in-service training is an integral part of successful provision of domiciliary dental care services (Merry and Edwards 2002).

It has been suggested that, if domiciliary dental care services are to evolve, dentists and dental hygienists must be aware and sensitive to the disabled person's needs. Therefore the dental team will need to develop appropriate communication styles and skills, be able to use their surgery-based clinical skills in the home-environment, maintain standards of infection control and personal safety (risk assessment) while remaining adaptable and flexible with regard to treatment goals, have a good knowledge of medical conditions and be able to deal successfully with medical emergencies. In addition the dental team must liaise and form informal referral networks with other primary care workers in order to provide domiciliary dental care services. Domiciliary care has been considered as an example of best practice as it increases access to care by reducing physical and emotional barriers and those associated with inequitable distribution of surgery-based dental services.

The British Society for Disability and Oral Health's document entitled 'The Development of Standards for Domiciliary Dental Care Services: Guidelines and Recommendations' (Fiske and Lewis 2000) has been published to provide a working framework for those undertaking domiciliary dental care. It defines domiciliary dental care services as:

> 'A service that reaches out to care for those who cannot reach the service themselves. The term domiciliary care is intended to include dental care carried out in an environment where a patient is resident either permanently or temporarily, as opposed to the care which is delivered in dental clinics or mobile units. It will normally include residential units and nursing homes, hospitals, day centres and the patient's own home.'

(Fiske and Lewis 2000)

and the aim as providing appropriate and accessible dental health care to all patients who for whatever reason are unable to attend and receive surgery-based care.

This document provides the practitioner with a planning and treatment schema for domiciliary dental care services. It includes a list of the types of patients requiring domiciliary dental care services, the knowledge and skills needed and detailed information on planning the visit, health and safety issues, planning treatment and the types of equipment (Table 4.15) which will be required. In addition, examples of domiciliary referral forms, recommended equipment data and costs are provided including an infection control policy for domiciliary dental visits (Fiske and Lewis 2000).

Integration of the dental team within the primary care team

Most of the publications dealing with the care of special needs patients insists upon teamwork. This has been emphasised within the dental team and for dental health professionals to undergo special needs awareness training together with continuing professional development to become skilled in the dental health care of special needs patients in the primary care setting. At the centre of this integrated care pathway is the patient and the carer with the emphasis being on patient-centred care. The need to use patient-centred

Table 4.15 British Society for Disability and Oral Health: Domiciliary care
(BSDOH Guidelines and recommendations 2000)

Domiciliary equipment

The equipment required will depend on the number and type of visits planned and the
resources available to purchase it. However, the following checklist may be helpful.
This list is an *aide memoire*, and is not prescriptive. Other items may be included according to individual preference. Some recommended items of equipment are listed
in Appendix 3.

General	Portable light	Portable suction
	Infection control items and equipment:	
	Gloves	Masks/Face visors
	Sharps disposal	Disinfection solution
	Liquid soap	Plastic over-sheaths/cling film
	Waste bags	Paper towels, rolls, tissues
	Dirty instrument-carrying receptacle	Protective spectacles for patient
	Laerdal resuscitation pocket mask	Emergency drugs kit/oxygen
	Protective clothing for dentist and nurse e.g. plastic aprons	
Administrative	Identification badge	Prescription pad
	Diary	BNF
	Appointment cards	Mobile phone
	Record cards	Pen
	Referral forms	A–Z Route Map
	Laboratory forms	Change for parking
	Post-op instruction leaflets	Medical history forms
	Consent forms	Health promotion literature
Prosthetic Kit	Impression material	Scalpel
	Impression trays and mixing equipment	Shade guide
	Safe air heater	Articulation paper
	Portable motor, handpieces and burs	Plastic bags
	Waxes	Gauze
	Pressure relief paste	Cotton wool rolls
	Bite registration material	Vaseline
	Wax knife	Denture fixative
	Bite gauge	Dividers
	Paint scraper/occlusal rim trimmer	Indelible pencil
Conservation kit	Portable unit (motor and suction)	Handpieces and burs
	Conservation instruments and tray	Light source
	Syringes, needles, needle-guards	Mirrors

(*Continued*)

Table 4.15 (continued) British Society for Disability and Oral Health		
Materials	Temporary dressing materials	Dry socket medicament
	Filling materials	Local anaesthetic cartridges
	Matrix bands	Topical anaesthetic cream/spray
	Gauze	Suture materials
	Cotton rolls and pellets	Haemostatic agents
	Vaseline	Bite packs
Periodontal kit	Hand scalers	Portable ultrasonic scaler
	Toothbrushes/pastes/therapeutic agents, e.g. Corsodyl, Omnigel	
Surgical kit	Forceps	
	Elevators	
	MOS Instruments including instruments for suturing	

strategies to elicit the patient's and/or carer's needs paves the way for joined-up dental health care.

Research has pointed to the urgency to recognise 'joined-up' health care provision between various primary care agencies. As special needs patients do not seem to self-refer for dental care, despite often having poor oral health; they remain unseen and apparently neglected. The need to integrate and connect with other primary care workers would allow the provision of seamless health care. This has been recognised as a priority by the Royal College of Surgeons (2001). However 'joined-up' or seamless health care is dependent upon informal networks between health professional groups so allowing the promotion of cross-referrals from community nurses or social workers to dentists working in the primary care setting (Smith and Freeman 2003).

4.3 ASSESSING PEOPLE WITH SPECIAL DENTAL NEEDS

The skills to assess those with special needs who can be treated with ease in the dental surgery are similar to those described in the Chapter 2 concerning the assessment of those with dental anxiety. The need to use appropriate communication skills and to listen carefully to the patients' history will provide the basis of the assessment process.

In a series of guidelines and recommendations from the British Society for Oral Health and Disability they describe the pathway that dentists must use when assessing patients with special needs. The Royal College of Surgeons' (2001) report identifies areas of good practice, in this regard, and lists a series of recommendations ranging from communication skills, oral health promotion to the education of parents, carers and professionals for those caring for people with learning disability. However, an additional communication skill is required for those with special dental needs and that is in relation to informed consent. It is necessary to use words and language that patients may understand in order to ensure that they have given their consent to treatment. The recommendations from both the British Society for Oral Health and Disability Recommendations and Guidelines and the Royal College of Surgeons set the adult and/or child with special needs in the dental practitioners' dental surgery. These documents provide support for the Disability Discrimination Act (DfES 1995) and NHS dentistry: Options for Change (DH 2002) as the guidelines and recommendations state that primary dental services must be accessible for all. The requirement remains for dentists to identify those who can be treated with dignity in their dental surgeries and those for whom secondary level care will afford acceptable and appropriate oral health care.

Patients with learning disability (Griffiths et al. 2000)

The Royal College of Surgeons (2001) has proposed a series of models of integrated service provision for people with learning difficulties. In each of these models (fig. 4.8) the dental team forms part of the integrated care programme. Integrating dental care services within the primary care sector provides a means by which primary dental services can be responsive and accessible to all patients who wished to use them. In addition patients with specific dental treatment needs can be identified with appropriate and accessible oral care provided. The need for referral for secondary level care can be clarified and steps taken to provide acceptable and affordable dental treatment.

While it is accepted that traditionally those who care for patients with special needs tend to be medical practitioners there has been a shift with the main providers of health care being those within the community setting. For patients with mental health problems community-based health care has formed 'the cornerstone' (Griffiths *et al.* 2000) of service delivery. Primary health care services for those with learning disability are perceived as equivalent, with dental practitioners providing one spoke of the primary care wheel by delivering services in the community setting. At the centre of the wheel of integrated care is the patient with primary health and social services providing the support to improve the oral health experiences for those with learning disability.

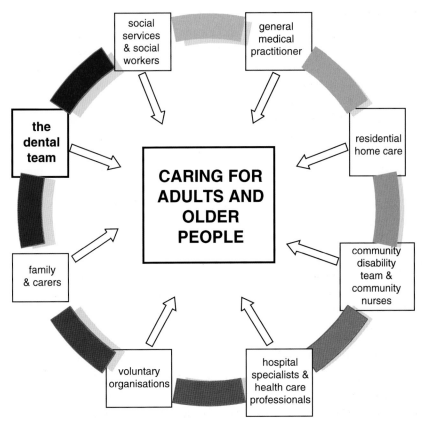

Figure 4.8 Integrated care for adults and older people with special needs (Royal College of Surgeons 2001).

Patients with mental illness

The patients most likely to be encountered and treated in the surgery setting are those residing in their own homes, in residential care or those who are homeless. These patients may have a series of behavioural difficulties which may limit their ability to accept the dental treatment which is being offered and provided. Factors which may limit the formation of a treatment alliance include the patient's mood and anxiety, motivation and self-esteem; their habits, life-style and their ability to maintain their oral health (Griffiths *et al.* 2000). In addition the patient's oral health status may be such that it is not possible to provide the desired treatment. It is essential therefore that dentists use their communication and clinical skills so that they can recognise and assess patients with mental health problems in order to provide appropriate and acceptable patient-centred primary dental services.

In the 'Oral Health Care for People with Mental Health Problems: Guidelines and Recommendations', Griffiths *et al.* (2000) provide the practitioner with a document which has been written for use in primary dental care. The recommendations are couched within the dental clinical arena while the appendices provide information with regard to psychiatric diagnostic categories, side-effects and oral side-effects of medication as well as self-help groups and organisations.

The first step in the assessment of the mentally ill patient is associated with the chronicity of their illness. It is often the case that patients in the prodromal phase of mental illness may first be seen by dental health professionals when they attend for treatment. It has been suggested that dentists have a role in identifying patients who may be in the early stages of mental illness. The range of mental health problems identified by dental practitioners include dental anxiety, low-spiritedness or depression and severe mental illnesses such as obsessive compulsive disorder or schizophrenia. The need to be able to identify and differentiate dentally phobic patients, who may have a more generalised psychological disturbance, from those with dental anxiety has been described elsewhere. However, there are other patients whose demands appear excessive and for whom dentists are concerned. These patients may present with excessive complaints or anxieties about the shape of their teeth, crowns or jaw and may be thought of descriptively as suffering from dysmorphophobia. These patients believe that part of their body is in someway deformed and their belief has the quality of a delusion. Particular care must be taken when the patient is an adolescent or in early adulthood because dysmorphophobia may be a prodromal symptom of schizophrenia. When presented with patients such as these the dental practitioner must refer to their medical colleagues for psychiatric secondary level care.

The second step is to make an assessment of the patients' oral health needs as patients may present with a series of oral health problems which on the one hand may indicate mental disturbance and on the other hand be a consequence of medication and/or neglect. Oral health symptoms include, tooth erosion, xerostomia and rampant caries. Tooth erosion is commonly observed in patients with anorexia nervosa and bulimia. Interestingly the tooth surface affected can indicate diagnosis as it tends to be the palatal and lingual-occlusal surfaces that are eroded in patients who vomit whereas the buccal surfaces are affected in those who do not.

Xerostomia is often observed in patients with mental illness and may be a consequence of dehydration (as in those with bulimia), taking prescription drugs (such as antidepressants or tranquilisers) or using illicit drugs. Patients with dry mouths have greater difficulty in speaking, chewing and swallowing and managing dentures. In addition they are more prone to dental caries, periodontal disease and oral infections.

Rampant caries is associated with xerostomia and is often an indicator of injecting drug use. Injecting drug users have the propensity to have a diet high in sugars and poor oral hygiene and when this is combined with xerostomia rampant caries follows. The use of methadone syrup adds to the difficulties as this dries the mouth and is high in cariogenic sugars.

The third step is to contact the patients' other primary care providers including the general medical practitioner and community mental health team (Griffiths *et al.* 2000). Liaising with the patients' other carers will provide support for the patient and the dental team by providing information with regard to the patient being able to undertake the treatment which is being offered and provided.

Patients with physical disability

Using a similar format to assess patients with physical disability, Arnold *et al.* (2000) in the document 'Guidelines for Oral Health Care for People with a Physical Disability' define what is meant by a physical disability before describing the need for the physical accessibility to dental surgery facilities. They (Arnold *et al.* 2000) link this with the Disability Discrimination Act (DfES 1995) to illustrate the importance of accessible health care for all. The need for wheelchair accessible care forms the kernel of this document. However, the requirement for dental health professionals to have patient-centred care with regard to those who are sight and/or hearing impaired is also emphasised. The recommendations provide the practitioner with a code of best practice as they detail the necessity to liaise with health, social and voluntary agencies, to have accessible dental services (including domiciliary care), to identify dental health criteria necessary to promote and maintain oral health together with the need to provide dental health education support for the patient, family and carers. The appendices give information on oral health assessments, the adaptation of buildings and facilities as well as health and safety issues in the workplace.

In conclusion, this section has aimed to place the role of the general dental practitioner and his/her team as part of the primary health care team providing oral health advice and treatment for patients with special dental needs. The need to conform and comply with Government legislation in order to provide an integrated, seamless and accessible dental health service for those with special needs has been stressed. Nunn (2000) writing in 'Disability and Oral Care' distinctly states the position and the part that dental health professionals must play in the oral care provision for those with disability and impairment. It is perhaps, therefore, appropriate to leave the last words to her (Nunn 2000):

> 'people with impairments are increasingly raising their profile within society through advocacy and slowly changing attitudes on the part of the communities, bullied to an extent by slow-moving legislation. Increasing numbers of people with impairments mean that their needs can no longer be denied by [the] caring professions. The evidence that behaviour, well-being and appearance are improved by good oral care and thus social acceptability enhanced, is irrefutable. The dental team have a role and duty to provide that care'

5.0 TREATMENT OF DENTAL EMERGENCIES

Treatment of dental emergencies is not only an integral part of a caring professional's practising life but is central to good patient management in dental practice. Good handling of dental emergencies has been considered to be a practice builder (de St. Georges 1990), not only for regular attenders but also as a means of converting the non-attender or irregular attender to becoming a regular attender. Patients may reasonably expect to receive an early response to a request for an emergency care when the practice is contacted during normal working hours, or to have some means of contacting their dentist or his/her deputy outside normal practising times, at least until 10 pm. Since 1991, dentists operating within NHS Regulations in the UK have had a statutory requirement to see their emergency patients within specified time periods, these time periods varying in different areas. Means by which patients may contact their dentist include the use of mobile telephones, message pagers, answering machines by way of a message left on the practice answering machine. The message should be clear, with instructions, especially telephone numbers, being given slowly so that they may be easily written down by the patient. It could be considered to be good practice to keep a log-book of contacts made by patients requesting emergency treatment, and of the actions taken.

Out-of-hours emergencies were delegated to a third party by 46% of respondents to a survey of Manchester dentists in 1993 (Burke *et al.* 1994), the results of which also showed that the most common emergencies were lost filling, fractured posterior tooth, loose crown or bridge, and swelling. This study also showed that 77% of respondent dentists managed their emergency appointments by 'double booking', while 33% arranged specific slots, and 22% worked longer hours to see their emergency patients, e.g. by booking patients during lunchtime or after normal surgery hours. It is important that patients attending out of normal working hours are accompanied by a chaperon, or that the dentist provides a chaperon.

5.1 WHAT IS AN EMERGENCY PATIENT?

An emergency patient has been defined as one 'which will attend at any time' (de St.Georges 1990). This would appear reasonable, given that slots left for emergency appointments will generally be at the least busy times in the appointment book. However, the dictionary definition (above) does not account for the patient who has fractured an anterior tooth or lost a crown before an important meeting; such patients could be termed *urgencies* rather than *emergencies*. Such 'urgencies' are just as important to that patient as the acute abscess is to another.

5.2 DIAGNOSIS AND MANAGEMENT OF COMMONLY SEEN DENTAL EMERGENCIES

Problems related to teeth

Basic principles

The dental pulp has no proprioceptive innervation, therefore pain of pulpal origin will be difficult for the patient to localise, except by association, e.g. tooth fracture or loss of filling occurred just prior to the commencement of the pain. Conversely, pain which can be localised will almost always be periodontal (lateral or apical) in origin. There are a number of questions and diagnostic aids which may assist in pain diagnosis:

Diagnosis of pain (Nehammer 1985):

Where is the pain?
When was the pain first noticed?
Describe the pain.
Any associated swelling?
Does anything relieve it?
Under what circumstances does the pain occur?
Previous dental history – ? history of recent treatment, periodontal treatment, history of trauma.

Diagnostic aids:

Periapical and bitewing radiographs
Pulp tester
Cold (ethyl chloride) or hot (hot GP stick)
Periodontal probe
Percussion

Pulpal pain

Pulpal pain may be hyperaemia, pulpitis (reversible or irreversible), leading ultimately to pulpitis/periodontitis and pulp death, this ultimately leading to a chronic or acute dentoalveolar abscess.

(i) Hyperaemia

The patient will complain of pain on hot and cold, with the pain diminishing when the stimulus is removed. The symptoms of hyperaemia may be similar to those of exposed dentine, in which the patient experiences symptoms of sensitivity to hot and cold; among the causes of dentine exposure may be a defective restoration, caries or exposed root dentine or cementum. The latter may only be made as a diagnosis when other causes have been ruled out by radiographic examination if necessary.

Treatment: Reassurance in some cases. Others, remove cause, place dressing in cavity or treat sensitive dentine or cementum, definitive treatment such as new restoration or glass ionomer to cover exposed root, later.

The cracked tooth syndrome

This was first described 30 years ago, with symptoms being essentially similar to those associated with hyperaemia or pulpitis, but, additionally, the cracked cusp may be tender to percussion (in comparison to periodontitis in which the whole tooth will be tender) and a crack may be visible on examination or transillumination. Diagnosis may also be made by asking the patient to occlude on a 'bite stick' placed on each cusp individually. The cusp which contains the crack will be tender on closing.

It may be necessary to remove a restoration from the tooth to examine whether the crack extends from the exterior to the base of the cavity, and observe under transillumination.

Treatment: Removal of the fractured part may relieve symptoms; however, it should be remembered that teeth do not always crack in a manner which is amenable to treatment and some fractures may extend into the pulp or periodontal membrane. It has also been considered that the symptoms disappear if and when the fractured portion breaks away.

(ii) Pulpitis

Irritation of the pulp causes inflammation, and the level of response is dependent upon the severity of the irritant. If this is mild, a layer of reparative dentine may be laid down as a form of protection from further injury. A more severe injury may cause death of cells and further inflammatory changes will take place which could eventually lead to pulp necrosis. In the early stages, the tooth will be sensitive to hot and cold, but not tender to percussion; at this stage the pulpitis may be *reversible* and the tooth may respond to removal of the stimulus. Later, the tooth will be both sensitive to hot and/or cold, the pain may be spontaneous and may last for longer periods of time, and the tooth may also be tender to percussion as the pulpitis becomes a periodontitis. The only treatments available for this stage of (*irreversible*) pulpitis are extraction of the tooth or pulp extirpation. In some instances, the tooth may be difficult to anaesthetise, and the only form of treatment possible may be the opening of the pulp to relieve pressure symptoms and the placement of a Ledermix (Blackwell Supplies Ltd., Gillingham, Kent, UK) paste dressing. This material contains eugenol, a tetracycline derivative and a topical corticosteroid which may reduce inflammation; it is in situations in which there is a vital pulp which is proving difficult to anaesthetise that Ledermix is most appropriate. It is therefore an essential part of the armamentarium for the treatment of the dental emergency.

(iii) Periapical abscess

This condition results from progression of an acute apical periodontitis. Radiographs may show little change from normal, depending upon the duration of the condition, but the condition may progress radiographically to a widened periodontal space after 10–14 days and progress to a well-defined radiolucency. The tooth will be tender to percussion. In acute cases, the tooth will be exquisitely tender and extrusion from the socket may cause the tooth to be mobile. Later, in acute cases there may be a swelling over the root apex which may ultimately involve the soft tissues of the face. In chronic cases, diagnosis may be more difficult, but the tooth may be slightly TTP and slightly mobile. In cases in which the patient complains of pain only on HOT, pain is likely to be of periodontal origin.

Treatment is to achieve drainage via the root canal, or extraction if conservation of the tooth is contraindicated. However, before commencing RCT, it is essential that it is established that the crown of the tooth can be restored.

(iv) Miscellaneous complaints

Pain may be related to recent treatment (Tables 4.16 and 4.17).

Patients may also attend complaining of gingival problems, and lost crown or fractured tooth (Tables 4.18 and 4.19).

Materials for temporary dressing

The material used will depend upon the period for which the dressing has to last. If the next available treatment slot is more than 2 weeks away, the use of

---

Table 4.16 Pain following treatment

Problem	Treatment
Restoration in hyperocclusion	Relieve occlusion.
Pain following instrumentation	Reassure and re-assess.
Galvanic action – pain will be on contact between dissimilar metals, with the patient also often complaining of a metallic taste	Polish new restoration and/or apply copal ether varnish or layer of unfilled resin.
Pulp exposure. If the pulp is vital, a pulpitis may ensue.	Pulp capping or RCT
If a non-vital pulp exposure has been missed during cavity preparation, there is a possibility that the placement of a well-sealed new restoration may prevent drainage of exudate or pus with the consequent build-up of pressure and acute pain.	Open and clean root canal

Table 4.17 Pain following endodontic treatment

Problem	Treatment
Pain after sealing Restoration in hyperocclusion	Relieve occlusion
Overfilling	Attempt removal of filling: however, removal of an overextended root filling is not always successful – apical surgery may be required if symptoms persist or if there are radiographic signs of infection.
Underfilling or inadequate debridement	Repeat root filling, control acute phase with antibiotics if necessary.
Root fracture	Extraction may be indicated, depending on site of fracture.
Pain following pulp extirpation is usually as a result of incomplete pulp removal or failure to properly instrument and debride the canal(s).	Spend time on proper instrumentation of the root canal(s)

polycarboxylate or glass ionomer may be advisable. If the waiting time for the next appointment is only days, the use of easily removed materials such as AZE may be appropriate. If the temporary dressing is ultimately to be replaced by a composite or amalgam restoration, glass ionomer may be indicated as this may ultimately be used as a base for the definitive restoration.

Lost provisional restoration

The construction of functional and aesthetically good provisional crowns or inlays is an important aspect of restorative dentistry. Such restorations, once called temporary restorations, are required to protect the tooth during the time from preparation/impressioning to return of the crown from the laboratory and the fit appointment. However, the fact that they are only required to function, in general, for a period of 1 to 2 weeks does not mean that they should be constructed without proper care and attention. A lost or fractured provisional restoration generates an emergency appointment, which is a waste of the dentist's surgery time, notwithstanding the time, inconvenience and, sometimes, irritation caused to the patient. The provision of aesthetically good, and functional provisional restorations is therefore of considerable importance. The construction of these restorations should therefore not be rushed at the end of the preparation visit. There is an advantage in

Table 4.18 Gingival and soft-tissue related problems

Problem	Treatment
Acute ulcerative gingivitis	by oral hygiene instruction, Chlorhexidine mouthwash, Metronidazole (Warning: side effects with alcohol), appointment for hygiene.
Pericoronitis associated with third molar tooth or erupting tooth in child patient	by Hot Salt Mouth Washes, antibiotics if necessary, appointment for removal of flap, removal of opposing tooth, or affected tooth.
Soft tissue swelling	by antibiotics for acute abscess, establishment of drainage if possible, arrange appointment for full diagnosis - ? lateral or apical
Aphthous ulceration. Possible cause, Toothbrush trauma – enquire if new toothbrush has been purchased, or, non-specific	by application of Orabase, avoidance of spicy foods, avoid area while brushing.
White slough next to carious cavity. Potential diagnosis, Aspirin burn; Patients may hold aspirin next to painful tooth in the hope that that will bring comfort, but this is not appropriate as aspirin is not absorbed through gingival tissue or oral mucosa.	by advice that this treatment is not appropriate. Keep area clean

constructing the provisional restoration before the impression is taken, namely, that the thickness of the restoration may be measured with callipers, which will provide a reading of the occlusal and labial reduction achieved. If this is considered insufficient, further reduction may be undertaken prior to impressioning. Shillingburg (1997) has described seven factors which should be satisfied with a good provisional restoration:

- Pulpal protection
- Positional stability, to prevent movement in a mesial/distal or occlusal direction
- Occlusal function – the provisional should provide occlusal harmony
- Easily cleaned
- Non-impinging margins
- Strength and retention – fracture of a provisional restoration may occur as a result of poor material choice, inadequate tooth preparation or incorrect occlusal adjustment leading to the provisional being in hyperocclusion

Table 4.19 Lost crowns and fractured teeth

Problem	Treatment
Lost crown. Causes of lost crown include traumatic occlusion, insufficient retention, dissolution of luting material, or, for post crown, root fracture	by recementation, having first checked (for post crowns) that there is no root fracture. Where there is insufficient retention, remake, or remake following crown lengthening surgery, may be appropriate.
Lost crown, where dentine core has fractured within the crown. Such cases are a scheduling nightmare, as the patient will have phoned for an emergency appointment, stating that they had lost a crown.	by removal of the dentine from the crown, preparing and placing a custom post (for root filled teeth) or root filling and placing a custom post (for vital teeth) and replacing the crown using chemically curing resin composite to fill the inside of the crown.
Fractured cusp(s) – MOD restorations are frequently implicated in cusp fracture in posterior teeth	by placing a glass ionomer dressing which will bond to tooth structure and mechanically adhere to the amalgam restoration
Fractured incisal corners	by placing a definitive restoration in resin composite

- Aesthetics – provisional restorations should be aesthetically satisfactory when these are placed in positions which are visible

  Choice of technique for provisional restorations for crowns and inlays

  The replica technique, in which a pre-operative impression is taken of the tooth to be prepared (or a wax up of it if the tooth is broken down) and those adjacent to it, holds a number of advantages over the use of pre-formed crowns:

- the occlusion on the provisional should more readily replicate that on the prepared tooth pre-operatively
- the shape of the provisional should replicate that of the prepared tooth pre-operatively, or its wax-up
- materials designed for use in the replica technique (such as Protemp Garant 3:3M ESPE, St.Paul, MN, USA) generally are available in a range of shades
- a more accurate marginal fit may be obtained by using the replica technique

  Laboratory-made provisional restorations may be of value if these restorations are required to last for longer periods of time. A pre-operative impression is cast, the dentist prepares the teeth on the plaster cast, the laboratory constructs the crowns in acrylic or a similar material and the clinician relines these at the chairside.

Surgical emergencies

A text on oral surgery should be consulted for a more complete exposition of these problems. Most common surgical emergencies are:

Problem	Treatment
Post-extraction bleeding	initially by application of pressure and suturing wound
Dry socket	by dressing, or antibiotics if wound closed.

Table 4.20 Summary of pain diagnosis

Where is the pain?
When was the pain first noticed?
Describe the pain
Is there any swelling?
Does anything relieve it?
What brings it on?
Any previous dental injuries or trauma?

REVERSIBLE PULPITIS; CAUSES
Caries
Fractured restoration or tooth
Exposed dentine
Trauma

PULPAL EMERGENCIES PRIOR TO TREATMENT
Pulpitis
Acute apical abscess
Cracked tooth syndrome

REVERSIBLE PULPITIS
Pain of short duration
Tooth not TTP
Pain difficult to localise
Exaggerated response to vitality testing
Radiographs – apex NAD

IRREVERSIBLE PULPITIS
Spontaneous bouts of pain
H & C bring prolonged pain
Pain may radiate

(*Continued*)

Table 4.20 (continued) Summary of pain diagnosis

Tooth may be TTP in later stages
Widened periodontal ligament in later stages

CRACKED TOOTH SYNDROME
Pain on chewing
One cusp may be TTP
Sensitivity to H & C
Pain may be difficult to localise

PAIN DURING TREATMENT
Restoration high in occlusion
Microleakage
Pulpal micro-exposure
Thermal injury
Mechanical injury
Chemical irritation
Galvanism
Stressed cusps due to one-increment curing of composite

6.0 REFERRALS

It is the sensible dentist who knows his/her limitations, and it is therefore beholden to the general dental practitioner to refer patients for whom s/he feels that treatment could be carried out to a higher standard, or more efficiently and effectively, to a specialist. It is not appropriate to refer a patient for financial reasons alone. In the NHS 'Dental Contract' of October, 1990, there is permissive provision for referral in para. 5 'Where a dentist does not have the necessary facilities, experience or expertise to provide the care and treatment required by a patient on his continuing care or capitation list, he may refer the patient to another GDP.' The General Dental Council is quite specific regarding referrals. In the May 2000 revision of 'Maintaining Standards' Para. 3.3 reads *'When accepting a patient a dentist assumes a duty of care which includes the obligation to refer the patient for further professional advice or treatment if it transpires that the task in hand is beyond the dentist's own skills. A patient is entitled to a referral for a second opinion at any time and the dentist is under an obligation to accede to the request and to do so promptly'*.

As patients often choose their GDP on the basis of convenience of travel to the surgery, a referral should be fully discussed with the patient in terms of ease of attendance, as well as cost, risks and potential for a successful outcome. The patient will then be able to make an informed decision on whether to agree to the referral and, if so, to decide the questions that they will ask the specialist.

6.1 RESPONSIBILITY OF THE REFERRING DENTIST

Responsibility for making an appropriate referral lies with the referring dentist, as an inappropriate referral is a waste of the specialist's time, let alone the inconvenience to the patient. Notwithstanding this, however, only a quarter of referrals to a unit of conservative dentistry were considered wholly appropriate when assessed by a peer group of GDPs (Burke *et al.* 1999).

The referral letter should be dated, should ideally be typewritten and signed by the referring dentist. It should contain the following:
- Name, address, date of birth and telephone number of the patient
- The patient's relevant dental and medical history
- A brief history of the patient's complaint and specific needs
- Whether the patient is being referred for treatment, advice or a second opinion
- The degree of urgency of the referral
- Whether the referral is for treatment under the NHS or privately, and, if the latter, Whether the patient is covered by appropriate private insurance
- The referring dentist's contact details

If appropriate radiographs of good quality have been taken, ideally these should be sent with the referral letter, with a request that they are returned at the earliest convenience. This prevents the need for the specialist to re-irradiate the patient.

6.2 RESPONSIBILITY OF THE SPECIALIST DENTIST

The specialist, on accepting a referral, must only undertake the treatment for which the referral was made. If additional treatment is indicated, this must be discussed with the patient and the referring dentist. Upon acceptance of the referral, the specialist should undertake the following:
- Contact the patient and provide directions, such as a map, to the practice or hospital.
- Explain, at the consultation appointment, what treatment, or alternative is proposed, its potential for success, and its cost.
- Discuss when payment should be made
- Obtain informed consent from the patient
- Ensure that arrangements are in hand for the patient's emergency care, if needed
- Write to the referring dentist either following the consultation with a treatment plan, or whenever treatment is completed

No financial incentives should be paid to encourage referrals.

Diplomatically expressed ethical guidance on referral can be found in the Medical Defence Union guide (Medical Defence Union, 1992):

> 'The dentist should bear in mind that for the benefit of patients all possible treatments should be made available with, if necessary, the assistance of other qualified dental or medical colleagues'.

6.3 REFERRAL FOR SPECIALIST ORTHODONTIC ASSESSMENT AND/OR TREATMENT (ANDREW RICHARDSON)

In UK, referrals can be to a Consultant in the hospital service, to a specialist practitioner or to an orthodontist in the Community Service. In general, specialist practitioners welcome referrals for treatment whereas Consultants receive referrals for treatment or advice. Most patients requiring combined treatments such as orthodontic appliances and surgery are treated by Consultants in hospitals. Patients in this category are easily recognised by their gross skeletal discrepancies and are frequently referred to Consultants either directly or through specialist practitioners.

In 1993 the European Commission Advisory Committee on the training of dental practitioners recommended that undergraduate training should include 'carrying out orthodontic corrections of minor occlusal problems' and 'knowing when to refer patients with more complex problems' (European Commission 1993).

When treatment in general practice of an assumed 'minor occlusal problem' proves more complex than expected, the practitioner will have no difficulty in recognising the need for referral. However, doubts have arisen over the recognition and appropriate stage of development for referral of more complex cases.

It has been considered that over 40 per cent of referrals are inappropriate and waste time because the patients are too young for treatment, because the malocclusions are too trivial, or that the patients are insufficiently motivated and have a level of mouth hygiene and dental decay which is incompatible with appliance therapy (Fox and Thompson 1993, O'Brien *et al*. 1996). Asking GDPs to be more selective in their referrals is an obvious next step. How this may be achieved is a point for discussion, but a cut-off point using the index of orthodontic treatment need (IOTN) has been proposed (Brook and Shaw 1989).

Of course, much depends on what is understood by the term 'orthodontic treatment'. If it means routine treatment of crowding or moderate inter-arch discrepancies with fixed appliances, the patient should be motivated and compliant, have a caries-free dentition, a high standard of mouth hygiene and eruption of all teeth back to the second molars. This implies that the patient is aged over 12 years.

Guidelines for referral can be found in the use of indices or 'triggers', in British Orthodontic Society (BOS) recommendations.

The Department of Health in the UK has proposed that access to orthodontic treatment under the NHS should require an IOTN score of 4 or above for the dental health component (Table 4.21) with the threshold falling to 3 (Table 4.22) when the Aesthetic Component (Table 4.23) is 6 or above. Indices are particularly appropriate at the later stage of dental development, for example, after 12 years.

Table 4.21 IOTN Dental health component grade 4 or above

The most striking occlusal abnormality in the patient is compared with the following list:
- Impeded eruption of teeth (except for third molars).
- Hypodontia with orthodontic and/or restorative implications.
- Overjet greater than 6 mm.
- Reverse overjet greater than 3.5 mm or 1 mm in the presence of masticatory and speech difficulties.
- Cleft lip and palate and other cranio-facial anomalies.
- Submerged deciduous teeth.
- Anterior or posterior crossbites with greater than 2 mm discrepancy between retruded contact position and intercuspal position.
- Posterior lingual crossbite with no functional occlusal contact in one or both buccal segments.
- Severe contact point displacements greater than 4 mm.
- Extreme lateral or anterior open bites greater than 4 mm.
- Increased and complete overbite with gingival or palatal trauma.
- Partially erupted teeth, tipped and impacted against adjacent teeth.
- Presence of supernumerary teeth.

Table 4.22 IOTN Dental health component grade 3

The most striking occlusal abnormality in the patient is compared with the following list:
- Overjet greater than 3.5 mm but less than or equal to 6 mm with incompetent lips.
- Reverse overjet greater than 1 mm but less than or equal to 3.5 mm.
- Anterior or posterior crossbites with greater than 1 mm but less than or equal to 2 mm discrepancy between retruded contact position and intercuspal position.
- Contact point displacements greater than 2 mm but less than or equal to 4 mm.
- Lateral or anterior open bite greater than 2 mm but less than or equal to 4 mm.
- Deep overbite complete on gingival or palatal tissues but no trauma.

Table 4.23 Aesthetic component 6 and above

The Aesthetic Component consists of a scale of 10 colour photographs showing different levels of dental attractiveness (Evans and Shaw 1987). Grade 6 shows retroclined upper central incisors, a proclined upper lateral incisor which is spaced from the central and some crowding of a lower canine tooth. The irregularity in the patient need not correspond precisely to the illustration but should have a similar cosmetic detriment.

Triggers

Kirschen (1998) has proposed a screening system to identify those children who would benefit from referral to an orthodontist. The chief advantage of the Kirschen system is that the screening can be done in less than a minute. The screening at age 9 years consists of 5 clinical triggers for further investigation. These are:

- **Delayed eruption** as judged by an abnormal sequence or comparison with the contralateral side.
- **Crowding** as judged by overlapping teeth or lateral incisors almost in contact with first deciduous molars.
- **Overjet** which exceeds 4 mm.
- **Crossbites.**
- **Submergence** of deciduous molars.
  Recommended additional triggers not included in the 60 second screening are:
- **Caries** with particular reference to carious or hypoplastic first molars or early loss of deciduous canines or molars.
- **Deep overbite or open bite** which are not included in the one minute examination because it is likely that they would be found in conjunction with another trigger.
  A further additional trigger appropriate at age 12 is:
- **Palpation for unerupted canines**. The patient should be referred if the maxillary canines are not palpable in the buccal sulcus.

British Orthodontic Society (BOS) guide (1996)

The BOS in its 'Young practitioner guide to orthodontics' recommends possible referrals at 3 stages of development:

(i) Deciduous to mixed dentition stage
  - Delayed eruption of permanent incisors.
  - Supplemental incisors when unsure which to extract.
  - Hypodontia.
  - Two or more upper incisors in crossbite.
  - Impaction of one or more first permanent molars.

- Severe crowding.
- Severe skeletal discrepancies – especially Class II.

(ii) Late mixed dentition
- Severe skeletal problems.
- Unfavourably positioned canines or other teeth.
- Hypodontia.
- Poor quality first permanent molars or other teeth of poor prognosis where timing of extractions may simplify subsequent treatment.

(iii) Early Permanent dentition
- Severe skeletal problems, including those where functional appliances may be indicated.
- Patients with unerupted teeth of doubtful prognosis, especially impacted canines.
- Uncertain choice of extraction patterns.
- Teeth which require rotation or bodily movement.

Referral for advice

In relation to referral for advice, the situation is widely variable. In some regions, Consultants make time to see almost all patients who are to be treated by practitioners (or at least their study casts and radiographs). Others prefer to place the emphasis on treatment by specialists who do not need advice so often. At the end of the day the best advice is for practitioners to get to know the Consultant and specialists in their region. They will usually have an established policy on giving advice.

6.4 REFERRALS FOR ORAL SURGERY AND ORAL MEDICINE (GRAHAM R OGDEN)

As with any other dental discipline, the need to refer will be governed by:
(a) the experience of the surgeon,
(b) the facilities available to the surgeon, such as availability of equipment, and, suitably trained staff, and
(c) patient factors such as medical problems, or, poor cooperation.

In general, biopsy is best left to the specialist that will treat the case, particularly when malignant disease is suspected. However, any soft tissue removed during the course of routine treatment should be sent for biopsy, appropriately fixed. If sent through the post, it should be fixed in formalin, correctly sealed and labelled (e.g. 'pathological specimen – fragile with care' including the name and address of the sender) together with a suitable pathology specimen form.

Patient's reason for attendance

The issue under investigation may be divided into a hard tissue (tooth or bone) or soft tissue (e.g. mucosa, nerve tissue) problem. The history of the condition should be established by asking questions such as –
- 'How long has it been present?'
- 'What makes it better?'
- 'What makes it worse?'
- 'Are there any associated signs or symptoms?' 'If so, what are they?'
- 'Is it getting worse?'

For pain
- 'Where does it radiate to?'
- 'What is its character?'
- 'How long does it last for?'

Past medical history

As well as a standard medical history, of particular note for oral surgery is the need to identify:
a) allergy to medicines, particularly antibiotics (ensure you differentiate side effects such as stomach pain from allergy, for example, itchy rash),
b) conditions, such as specific heart disease, requiring prophylaxis against infective endocarditis;
c) previous radiotherapy to the orofacial region that might predispose to osteoradionecrosis after extractions;
d) any medicines, drugs, tablets being taken, particularly those prescribed by their doctor, e.g. Warfarin.
e) questions relevant to the risk of exposure to v CJD, such as human growth hormone received prior to 1985, or neurosurgical procedures, particularly those involving human dura mater prior to 1985.

Differential diagnosis

In the middle of a busy clinic, it can be difficult to recall all the possible causes, of, say, a swelling on the palate. The surgical sieve allows rapid consideration of potential causes when seeking to decide whether to refer a case or not. A couple of options can usually be recalled:
- Iatrogenic (you caused it!)
- Idiopathic (no one knows how it arose)
- Metabolic
- Tumour (Benign or Malignant)

- Infection (Viral, Bacterial, Fungal)
- Inflammatory (Acute, Chronic)
- Trauma
- Drug induced

Conditions which may require referral

Following is the majority of conditions in which referral may be considered appropriate:

Dental infection

- Any infection unresponsive to antibiotics, in which the dental cause cannot be removed.
- Infection that may compromise airway or swallowing.

Dental extraction

- Retained root / impacted tooth requiring > 30 minutes surgery time.
- Where GA is required.
- History of post extraction problems, e.g. persistent bleeding, oro-antral communication.
- Impacted teeth – where risk of morbidity is high, e.g. ID nerve involvement with wisdom teeth or where access is reduced.

Orthodontic assessment for impacted canines or developmental anomalies.

Special investigations

- Those not available such as panoramic radiography which may not be available in all practices.

Miscellaneous

- Where signs, such as swelling or pain have occurred and a dental cause has been excluded.

Mucosa

- Any oral mucosal lesion that fails to heal within 2 weeks in the absence of an obvious aetiological factor.

Neural disorders

- Unexplained sensory loss.

Facial palsy.

Hard tissue

- Jaw deformities
- Fractures of the facial skeleton
- Tumours
- Cysts – other than small lesions associated with non-vital teeth.

Additional reasons for referral include:

- Where a second opinion is sought, for example, at the patient's request or when GDP is uncertain of the diagnosis or treatment.
- Where the surgeon lacks experience or staff/equipment support

Assessment prior to referral

Space does not permit the presentation of a detailed guide on the investigations which should be undertaken for the conditions above, so, the assessment of impacted wisdom teeth – a common reason for referral from dental practice, and oral cancer – a condition of potential life-threatening importance, will be presented as examples.

Assessment of impacted wisdom teeth

It does not necessarily follow that because a tooth is impacted it has to be removed. In all cases, the patient should be aware of the various possible treatment options, including the potential consequences of NOT removing the impacted tooth. Panoramic radiographs or oblique lateral views are the radiographic views for assessment of wisdom teeth, as it can be difficult to obtain a satisfactory periapical view.

Criteria for removal of wisdom teeth

There have been a number of published guidelines (NIH, RCS England, SIGN, etc.) that include the following indications for removal of lower third molars:

- Pericoronitis
- Unrestorable caries in the third molar
- Caries in the distal of the lower second molar that cannot be adequately treated because the 3rd molar is in the way (fig. 4.9)
- Periodontal disease due to third molar impaction
- Pathology associated with the wisdom tooth
- Resorption of lower second molar due to the wisdom tooth

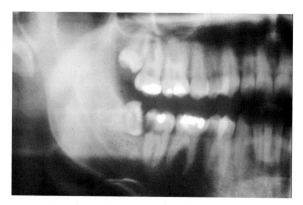

Figure 4.9 Horizontally impacted third molar associated with caries in the distal aspect of the lower second molar.

Criteria where removal of wisdom teeth is not deemed advisable include:
- patients whose third molars would be judged to erupt successfully and have a functional role in the dentition.
- patients whose medical history renders removal an unacceptable risk to the overall health of the patient or where the risk exceeds the benefit.
- patients with deeply impacted third molars with no history or evidence of pertinent localised systemic pathology.
- patients where the risk of surgical complications is judged to be unacceptably high or where fracture of an atrophic mandible may occur.
- Where the surgical removal of a single third molar tooth is planned under local anaesthesia, simultaneous extraction of asymptomatic contralateral teeth should not normally be undertaken.

Assessment of degree of difficulty in removing lower 3rd molars

Three methods can be used (fig. 4.10)
1. Type of impaction
2. Depth of impaction
3. Distance between anterior ramus and second molar

The need to refer will rely upon the surgeon's experience, equipment, type of impaction and patient factors, e.g. medical history. In general, refer those cases where a strong indication for removal exists in which the tooth is not vertically or mildly impacted. The most difficult impaction (thus best referred) are distoangular inclined wisdom teeth that are covered with bone in which there is limited space between the second molar and anterior ramus. It is also best to refer when the risk of morbidity is high.

Factors influencing morbidity
1. Position of ID canal. On a panoramic radiograph, deviation of ID canal, a dark band overlying root of 8, or a break in the white cortical line of the canal – all suggest that the root of the lower 3rd molar is involved with the ID canal.
2. Predisposition to infection, e.g. Smokers, Diabetics, immunologically suppressed patients.
3. Potential duration of operation
4. Use of antibiotics, steroids and oral hygiene to reduce infection and swelling.

All patients should be warned of pain, swelling, bruising, trismus and possible dysaesthesia to lip and tongue. In addition, factors influencing quality of life are important, e.g. diet and enjoyment of food and time off work.

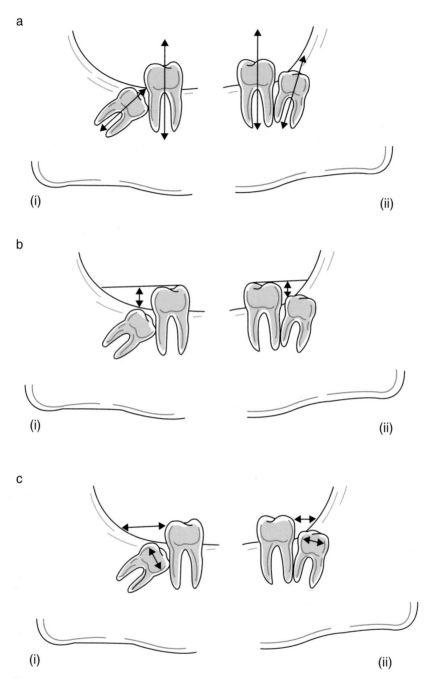

Figure 4.10 a) Orientation of third molar: (i) towards second molar; (ii) away from second molar. b) Increased depth of crown of right third molar (i) from occlusal plane compared to left third molar (ii). c) Distance between anterior ramus and distal aspect of second molar compared with width of third molar crown: increased surgical access for right third molar (i) but reduced access for left third molar (ii).

Oral cancer

Early signs

Early lesions which are referred and treated can significantly improve the prognosis for the patient. Symptoms (such as pain) are lacking. Although the full list of potentially malignant conditions should be appreciated, particular care should be taken in identifying any change in colour, particularly red or speckled (red/white) lesions (fig. 4.11). White lesions, e.g. keratosis, have a lower rate of malignant change but should be monitored, e.g. photograph and referred for biopsy. The general dental practitioner should:

Assess exposure to risk factors, e.g. smoking, excess alcohol, diet lacking fresh fruit/vegetables and previous upper aerodigestive cancer.

Note: Limits of safe drinking are 14 (female) and 21 (male) units/week. Excess intake (greater than 35/50 units (F:M)) is potentially damaging to health. A unit of alcohol is approximately equivalent to one glass of wine, half pint of beer, or a single measure of spirit ('short').

When the suspect lesion is first seen, record its dimensions in the patient's notes, together with its exact site and colour. Consider taking a photograph. Review in two weeks. If no improvement, then refer via telephone to arrange urgent opinion if necessary. Any lesion e.g. ulcer, present for more than 2 weeks, showing no sign of healing, should be considered malignant and referred urgently for biopsy.

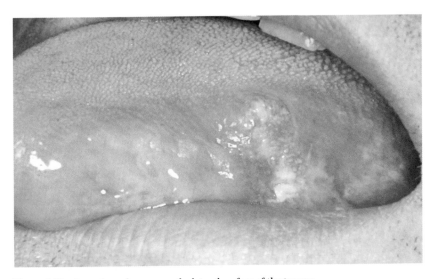

Figure 4.11 An early oral cancer on the lateral surface of the tongue.

Late signs

There may be sensory disturbance, (e.g. numb lip) or motor disturbance (e.g. deviation of tongue to affected side on thrusting tongue forward), dysphagia, weight loss and anaemia. In such cases, the tumour may have spread to the regional lymph nodes (e.g. hard, tethered).

Other conditions

There are a number of other conditions for which urgent referral and hospitalisation is indicated. These include:
Ludwig's angina (fig. 4.12).

In this condition, the patient will experience difficulty in swallowing and the airway may be compromised. There will be a bilateral submandibular

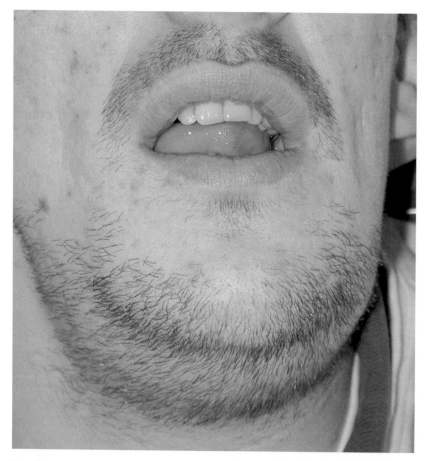

Figure 4.12 Ludwig's angina. Bilateral swelling of the sublingual and submandibula spaces giving rise to limited mouth opening and potentially compromising the airway.

swelling causing floor of mouth to be swollen and tongue enlarged. This is life threatening. An ambulance should be called if the airway is at risk.

Persistent bleeding

The site of the bleeding should be established – is it from hard tissue or soft tissue? For soft tissue primary bleeding, haemorrhage should arrest with pressure, sutures or application of proprietary haemostatic gauze. Secondary bleeding usually occurs > 48 hours after operation, due to infection. Referral is indicated if bleeding is persistent and unresponsive to local measures. In such cases there may be an underlying haemostatic deficiency, e.g. clotting factor or platelet defect.

Tuberosity fracture/Tooth removed

If the maxillary posterior tooth is removed with the tuberosity, check for oroantral communication. If there is bleeding or loose tissue, then suture.

Tooth retained in fractured tuberosity

If the reason for extraction is not infection, then consider splinting it, with surgical removal 3–4 weeks later. If the tooth is infected, then remove with bone and suture over defect.

Oroantral communication/fistula (OAF)

History: There will be loss of liquid from mouth out of the nose and a history of extraction of posterior maxillary tooth. Where extraction occurred on a previous day, confirm the antral communication by getting patient to pinch nose and attempt to breathe out through nose. Air will bubble around the socket of the extracted tooth. Radiographs are not always confirmatory due to superimposition of other bony structures, although they should show the proximity of the roots to the maxillary antrum.

Treatment is by referral to a specialist for a buccal advancement flap under LA. If small and noticed at the time of extraction, construct a coverplate to protect the socket and advise the patient to avoid blowing the nose/or sneezing for 2 weeks.

6.5 REFERRAL OF PATIENTS WITH TEMPOROMANDIBULAR DISORDERS (TMD) (ROBIN GRAY)

Preliminary patient assessment for TMD

The title 'Temporomandibular Disorders' (TMD) is a generic term and covers several diagnoses, the most common being pain dysfunction syndrome (PDS), also known (amongst other titles) as facial arthromyalgia.

Internal derangements (ID) of the temporomandibular joint (TMJ) are also commonly seen. These can present in one of two ways; firstly, and most often, as disc displacement with reduction (clicking) and, secondly, as disc displacement without reduction (locking).

The third TMD, which may be less frequently seen, is degenerative joint disease, usually osteoarthrosis (OA).

It should be remembered, however, that the TMJ may be involved in other systemic diseases such as rheumatoid arthritis and psoriatic arthritis but rarely, if ever, as the first joint involved.

Finally, the dentist may be called upon to see, as an emergency, the patient who has developed a TMD, usually a traumatic arthritis, as a result of trauma.

There are several other conditions that are included under the umbrella of the term 'TMD' such as developmental abnormalities, tumours and infection but these are very rarely encountered.

What are the diagnostic criteria?

The diagnostic criteria of the more common TMD are listed below:

Pain Dysfunction Syndrome (PDS)

- There is pain on palpation of the temporomandibular joint.
- There is pain or tenderness distributed throughout the areas of attachment of the mandibular muscles.
- There is limitation or deviation (usually toward the affected side) of mandibular movement.
- The symptoms are often worse on waking in the morning.
- Clicking may be a feature but is usually intermittent.
- Headache may also be a factor.

ID: Disc displacement with reduction

- Reciprocal clicking (clicking on opening and closing) which is constantly present.
- The opening click is usually louder than the closing click.
- There is usually a transient deviation towards the affected side.
- The click may or may not be painful.
- There may be acute TMJ pain when clenching the teeth due to compression of the innervated posterior parts of the disc.

ID: Disc displacement without reduction

- Limitation of mandibular movement (locking) due to a physical obstruction.
- There is usually a lasting deviation towards the affected side.
- The locking may or may not be painful.
- Locking is usually preceded by a history of clicking.

- At the onset of locking mandibular opening is usually limited to about 17–20 mm.
- With the passage of time mouth opening will improve slightly.

Osteoarthrosis
- There is pain usually localised to the area of the temporomandibular joint.
- The joint sound is crepitus.
- The symptoms usually are worse as the day goes on and with function.
- The muscles may not be tender.

Trauma
- The patient will present with a germane history and usually with pain in one or both joints.
- There may be limitation of movement and general, and possibly acute, tenderness of not only joints but also masticatory muscles.

Who are the patients liable to be?

Contrary to the popular belief that the symptoms of TMD are more common in females than males, they are, in fact, present in equal proportions in both sexes. It is a well-established fact that in all medical outpatient attendances more females than males present for treatment and it is this that accounts for the preponderance of females in patient studies.

In the overwhelming majority of TMD patients it is usually impossible to link the onset of symptoms to a specific event or aetiological factor. There are, however, some contributory factors that are often reported by the patients.

The symptoms of PDS are most commonly found in the younger age group – teens, 20s, 30s, – and may be associated with stressful life events. In addition, parafunctional activities such as bruxism and clenching are common.

While TMJ clicking is expected at some stage in life in over 50% of the population, the symptoms of ID are now becoming more frequently encountered in the younger age group. It is unusual for a patient to experience locking without a previous history of clicking.

The symptoms of OA are most often found in the older age group (50+ years).

Psychological aspects
It should be remembered that a group of 'TMD patients' does not exhibit the same psychological profile as do other dental outpatients. It is the profile, however, of a group of 'chronic pain sufferers'.

TMD patients, as a group, generally have a different response to psychological questionnaires such as the general health questionnaire (GHQ). This means that their treatment response and treatment expectations may not be what one would anticipate. These patients are not psychiatrically ill; it is rather that their symptoms have assumed such a part of their life that their psychological profile is altered. As treatment progresses and their symptoms resolve then their responses return to within the normal range.

What are the most common subjective complaints and what are the most common clinical findings?

The most common reason for a patient to seek treatment is pain.

The most common subjective complaint, however, is of clicking, usually from one TMJ rather than both. This has often been present for some time prior to the patient asking for advice.

The features that make the patient attend for advice are either the onset of pain or the onset of locking. They may often have put up with clicking or restricted movement for quite a period and frequently say 'they thought this was normal'.

The most common clinical finding is temporomandibular joint clicking. This is followed by mandibular muscle tenderness and then by TMJ tenderness.

Clinical examination of the articulatory system. TMJs, Muscles, Occlusion.

TMJS

The temporomandibular joints should be examined for tenderness, sounds and range of movement.

TENDERNESS

The joints should be palpated with gentle but firm digital pressure in the immediate pre-auricular area but also, more importantly, via the external auditory meatus (EAM). The little finger should be placed in the EAM and gentle anterior pressure should be applied. The patient can then be asked to slowly open and close the mouth. As the principal area of innervation of the disc and capsule is the posterior part, tenderness is more readily detected by this method.

Joint sounds are best elicited by use of a stethoscope, preferably a stereo-stethoscope. This is an instrument with one set of earpieces but with separate diaphragms, one to place over each TMJ. By this method not only can joint sounds be heard but also it is easier to tell which side is clicking or which side clicks first.

Range of movement
The range of movement should be measured in both the vertical and lateral dimensions.

The lower limit of normal in the vertical dimension is regarded as being 35 mm for females and 40 mm for males. The range of opening can be assessed using a vernier gauge measuring from incisal tip to incisal tip. The overbite need not to be excluded.

Ask the patient to move to each side and, using the incisal midlines as the baseline, thereby assess the maximum range of movement on lateral excursion. The lower limit of normal is regarded as 8 mm in either direction.

Whilst other assessment of the progress of the patient's condition or of their treatment is often at best subjective or qualitative, the range of mandibular movement is the only **measurable and quantitative** param-eter available to monitor their current state.

Assess the pathway of opening. If there is a disorder affecting one joint or one side of the articulatory system then deviation of movement is usually, if not always, towards the affected side.

Muscles

It is often advocated that a series of mandibular and accessory muscles should be included in an overall TMD examination not only for the presence of direct tenderness but also for the presence of trigger points.

In reality there is only a small group of muscles that are readily accessible for manual palpation. While it is accepted that other muscles should be examined if there is a clinical reason for doing so, the primary muscles which should be included in a routine articulatory system examination, include the masseter, temporalis and lateral pterygoid muscles.

All these are small muscles and the areas of tenderness are usually their origins and insertions rather than the body of the muscles. Some are available to direct palpation whilst others should be examined against resisted movement.

Masseter
The origin of the masseter should be examined by bi-digital palpation at its origin over the anterior two-thirds of the zygomatic arch and over its insertion over the outer surface of the angle of the mandible.

One finger should be placed inside the vestibule of the cheek and the opposing finger on the skin surface. The attachments of the muscle can then be gently compressed to determine whether there is tenderness. One side should be compared with the other.

Temporalis

The origin of the temporalis can be examined in the temporal fossa between the superior and inferior temporal lines. It is usually the anterior elevator fibres which are tender.

Lateral pterygoid

This muscle is inaccessible to digital palpation. Pressing a digit up behind the maxillary tuberosity merely compresses the pterygo-mandibular raphe, the superior constrictor or the buccinator and the buccal pad of fat. A more reliable method of examining this muscle is against resisted movement. One hand is placed on the crown of the head while the other is placed under the chin. The patient is asked to open the mouth and, once partially open, any further movement is resisted. If there is pterygoid spasm the patient will immediately experience pre-auricular pain or discomfort. Resisted vertical movement tests both sides at the same time. One side can be tested individually by again placing a hand on top of the head and the other to one side of the chin. The patient is then asked to move the mandible to the side against resistance and, if pterygoid spasm is present then discomfort will be felt in the contra-lateral side.

Occlusion

Comprehensive texts outlining the examination of occlusion can be found elsewhere: this section lists the occlusal parameters the dentist should be familiar with and should routinely examine.

- Does centric occlusion occur in centric relation? If it does not, where is the premature contact and what is the direction of the slide from centric relation to centric occlusion?
- Where is the anterior guidance of the mandible? Is there canine guidance, group function or neither?
- Are there posterior interferences to smooth lateral excursions of the mandible on the working side, the non-working side or both?
- If present do these interferences extend up to and beyond the canine cross over position?
- Is there freedom in centric occlusion?

Also included in the examination of the articulatory system should be an assessment of the clinical signs of bruxism. These include attrition of the teeth and the presence of unusual wear facets, fracture of teeth and/or restorations, sensitivity of teeth, scalloping of the lateral border of the tongue and ridging of the buccal mucosa.

Special tests

Radiographs are of limited value for a variety of reasons. The tissue layers covering the surfaces of the TMJ are fibrous tissue as is the intra-articular disc.

These, therefore, will not be visualised. As the TMJ is not a regular structure and as the condylar angle varies on an intra-individual as well as on an inter-individual basis, the joint space cannot be accurately assessed. There needs to be between 40% and 60% demineralisation before any radiographic evidence of erosion can be seen. The standard transcranial oblique lateral view only shows a small part of the surface area which, in fact, is the lateral pole of the condyle and the lateral rim of the fossa which is not the load bearing part of the joint where damage, if present, might be expected.

For all these reasons radiographs should only be used to confirm the clinical diagnosis and then, only when absolutely necessary.

What to treat in practice and how to do it

The most commonly encountered TMD seen in general dental practice will include pain dysfunction syndrome, internal derangements, osteoarthrosis and the results of trauma.

The majority of temporomandibular disorders will respond to a combination of counselling, physiotherapy, pharmacotherapy and splint therapy.

In a very small percentage of cases further more invasive treatment might be necessary such as manipulation of the mandible under a general anaesthetic. Such treatment, however, is the remit of the specialist clinic.

Counselling

This term implies explanation and reassurance. Explanation is a very important part of treatment. Patients are often totally unaware of, for instance, a parafunctional habit. If the dentist examines the patient intra-orally and sees ridging of the buccal mucosa or scalloping of the tongue then it may be possible to point out to the patient that they are grinding their teeth. This raises the patient's awareness of a hitherto unknown activity and may assist in its prevention.

Physiotherapy

Most TMD patients are suffering from a musculo-skeletal injury and physiotherapy is a much under-utilised treatment in their management.

If someone damages any joint such as their knee or shoulder in an accident, then probably the first clinician's advice they would seek is that of a physiotherapist. TMD patients are no different. An intensive course of physiotherapy early in the course of the disorder will be very beneficial.

The optimal regime is the use of megapulse, ultrasound or laser two to three times per week for three to four weeks. Less than twice a week will probably be of little benefit.

If the diagnosis is of an internal derangement then the physiotherapist should be discouraged from aggressive exercise or manipulation during the acute phase because of the danger of further damage to the displaced intra-articular disc.

'Self help physiotherapy' can include the use of alternating hot and cold compresses and non-steroidal anti-inflammatory gels applied directly to the skin overlying the joint, assuming there are no medical contra-indications.

Pharmacotherapy

The most commonly used drugs are analgesics, non-steroidal anti-inflammatory drugs (NSAID) and benzodiazepines. There has been suggestion in the past that tri-cyclic antidepressant drugs have a role, but, due to the patient's unpredictable response and to a lack of pharmacological rationale for such a prescription in the management of TMD patients, these are best avoided.

The patient, prior to seeking advice, will usually have tried a variety of common analgesics.

The most commonly prescribed NSAID is ibuprofen. The usual prescription is for 400 mg three times per day. Patients should be counselled that if they take ibuprofen on an 'as needed' basis it is only as effective as paracetamol. To maximise the anti-inflammatory effect it must be taken regularly for three to four days before a therapeutic level is reached.

Benzodiazepines, however, do have a pharmacologically recognised muscle relaxant effect and are very useful in the management of acute muscle spasm. This is best prescribed as the oral suspension and the patient can thus titrate his or her own dose to take as little as necessary as a once per day dose before going to sleep to achieve muscle relaxation.

Splint therapy

It is impossible to be prescriptive about splint therapy within the remit of this section and again the reader is encouraged to consult a specialist text. There are four commonly prescribed appliances.

The soft poly-vinyl vacuum formed appliance is probably the most commonly provided. These appliances do have a role to play but usually only as short-term emergency appliances. It should be recognised that in a percentage of patients these appliances will exacerbate the symptoms because the patient is so aware of having something compressible in their mouth that it will encourage parafunction.

The localised occlusal interference splint is a useful device, which, by intentionally interfering with the patient's centric occlusion, will discourage parafunction. If the patient is bruxing in an extreme lateral excursion, however, this appliance will be ineffective.

The anterior repositioning appliance is an extremely beneficial appliance in the treatment of the internal derangement of disc displacement with reduction if it can be demonstrated at the chairside that the click disappears when the patient opens from and closes into a protruded mandibular position.

This appliance guides the mandible downwards and anteriorly to a position recorded by the dentist at which point the trauma to the anteriorly displaced disc is removed. This appliance appears to assist the disc to reposition.

The stabilisation splint is used when it appears there is a significant occlusal input into the patient's symptoms. This appliance provides all the features of an ideal occlusion with the provision of centric relation occlusion, anterior guidance on anterior teeth and elimination of posterior interferences.

It is not always necessary to treat all symptoms in all patients all of the time. The patient may be content to endure a long-standing click if their presenting complaint of pain, for example, is resolved.

Treatment should be approached on a threshold concept. The patient has the same joints, muscles and teeth they had prior to the onset of their symptoms in the overwhelming majority of cases. What the dentist should aim for is to 'tip' the patient back below this threshold whereby they continue to function with the same articulatory system they had before, but without symptoms.

The combination of treatments described above will result in alleviation of symptoms in approximately 85–90% of patients.

Second phase irreversible alteration to the patient's permanent dentition is usually not needed and is therefore best avoided.

Who to treat in practice and who not to treat in practice

The overwhelming majority of TMD patients can be successfully treated by the modalities outlined in the previous section and it is important to realise that the patient's general dental practitioner is probably best placed to manage the majority of cases as they know the individual and therefore know the treatment needs and expectations.

As has already been mentioned, however, there are differences in the 'TMD' group of patients from other attenders. There may well be significant underlying factors of which the clinician is unaware. With some patients it must be accepted that there will be no simple mechanical cure.

If the symptoms appear exaggerated in relation to what would be expected from the clinical findings, or if treatment is not proceeding as would have been anticipated (i.e. 'everything you do is making matters worse!'), then referral should be considered.

Who to refer. Who to refer to. How to refer

Referral to a colleague for a second opinion, referral for advice and delivery of a practice-based treatment plan, referral to someone in a different discipline for assistance in a patient's management or, if the clinical situation is out with one's experience, referral for all further management, are all options that should not be forgotten.

If there is doubt about the initial diagnosis but the patient and the dentist wishes the treatment to be carried out in the practice, then an option would be to refer the patient to a specialist for a **practice-based** treatment plan. There is little use in referring a patient in these circumstances if the treatment plan provided is not practical for either the dentist to undertake or the patient to finance.

Historically the only referral center for the GDP, if there was not ready access to a Dental Hospital, was the local Oral Surgery Unit. Nowadays, however, it is recognised the treatment of TMD is principally non-surgical and there are usually specialist practitioners locally with a particular interest.

If referral is necessary for assistance in treatment such as to a physiotherapist, then referral can be done either directly to the physiotherapy unit of the local hospital or via the patient's doctor. Often general medical practitioners will have direct access to the community physiotherapy services.

It is important to remember not to 'refer and forget'. It is the dentist's responsibility to monitor their patient's progress, possibly needing to intervene if they or the patient are not happy with the treatment received upon referral.

Headache

Dentists are, with increasing frequency, being asked to treat patients with headache. It has been reported in the literature that patients who are under treatment for a TMD and who also have headache as one of their symptoms, may experience resolution of the headache as their TMD improves. Other studies have investigated headache patients with no TMD experience and have treated them with occlusal splints and have found encouraging results.

One word of caution: Headache is a symptom not a disease and the correct clinician to make the initial diagnosis of headache is a neurologist not a dentist.

There is only **one headache** which dentists are qualified to diagnose and therefore to treat, namely, TMD related headache. This is:

> 'Chronic tension type headache associated with a disorder of the pericranial muscles where oro-mandibular dysfunction is a likely causative factor'.

Dentists may be part of the group of clinicians who treat headache but should not adopt the mantle of 'clinician in charge' in isolation and without reference to colleagues.

Conclusion

Many TMD patients may be successfully treated in general dental practice, with simple methods available to all clinicians, but some are better referred. Dentists should be aware of their knowledge and limitations, and the patient's expectations. Avoid irreversible change whenever possible. A combination of treatments is often best.

6.6 REFERRAL OF PATIENTS WITH TOOTH SUBSTANCE LOSS (TSL)

Although there is little published data on the incidence of tooth wear, also known as tooth substance loss, there is anecdotal evidence that patients are increasingly presenting with TSL and related problems. In general, the TSL which affects the younger age groups tends to be erosive, as a result of over-consumption of carbonated beverages, while in the older age groups, TSL is more likely to be multifactorial, involving erosion, abrasion and attrition. A management priority must be removal of the cause, and this will involve counselling the patient once the causative factors have been identified. However, in cases of erosive TSL when the patient is bulimic, counselling may be difficult, as the patient may not, at the outset, admit to their bulimic habit. In this respect, it has been considered that bulimia or other gastric reflux habits, may account for a substantial proportion of cases presenting with severe tooth substance loss in which the patient does not admit to dietary factors such as excessive consumption of citrus drinks or fruits, or carbonated beverages.

Treatment of TSL may be indicated for a variety of reasons. Patients may request treatment for a variety or reasons:
- because of poor aesthetics of chipped and worn teeth.
- because of sensitivity
- because of pain or infections associated with teeth which have become non-vital as a result of severe TSL
- because of reduced masticatory function
- because of difficulties in phonation
  Treatment may also be suggested by a dentist for a variety of reasons:
- because the TSL is progressing and the dentition requires protection by restorations from further TSL.
- because reduced function, TMJ disease or compromised aesthetics has been noted.

The patient may be unaware of the problem because of its slow rate of progression and it is sometimes the patient's partner or relative who draws attention to the TSL because of the worsening appearance of the patient's dentition. In general, therefore, except in cases of erosive TSL in young patients, treatment can be planned at a gentle pace.

6.7 HISTORY TAKING FOR PATIENTS WITH TSL

Prior to consideration of referral, a full history and complete examination should be carried out with the aim of making a definitive and accurate diagnosis (Watson and Burke, 2000). Details of the patient's concerns and symptoms should be obtained and of their duration and severity. A complaint of sensitivity to cold and hot may indicate rapid loss of tooth substance, as secondary dentine is not being laid down as quickly as the tooth substance loss is occurring. In such cases, early intervention may be indicated before the pulp becomes irreversibly damaged. Chipping of incisal enamel is another factor that patients may notice. The presence of these factors in the patient's history may provide a measure of how quickly the TSL is progressing. Most commonly, the patient's presenting complaint will be of poor aesthetics relating to shortened teeth, incisal translucency or chipping, functional problems such as difficulty in chewing, or sensitivity.

During history taking, an attempt should be made to guage the level of the patient's concern regarding his/her TSL, given that a patient who is unaware of their dental problems may be unlikely to undertake an extensive course of treatment. In such cases, the problems relating to TSL should be explained to the patient and an appointment made to review the patient's attitude. It should be remembered that a treatment option is no treatment – no-one dies from TSL!

The patient's medical history, with special reference to medical conditions which may predispose to gastric regurgitation, such as gastric ulceration, hiatus hernia, oesophagitis, and, gastro-oesophageal reflux should be taken. The patient should also be asked about indigestion or heartburn, both of which may indicate a tendency for gastric reflux. Pregnancy may indirectly be associated with TSL, given the possibility of repeated vomiting as a result of morning sickness. Similarly, excessive alcohol consumption may result in vomiting and/or gastritis, both of which could be contributory factors to TSL.

Some medications, such as chewable vitamin C, hydrochloric acid for achlorhydria and some iron-containing preparations, may predispose to TSL. Diets high in citrus fruits may also predispose to TSL, as too may diets which are high in carbonated beverages such as cola drinks. Some patients, in the younger age groups, may 'swish' the carbonated drink around their mouths. It could be considered that this would increase the overall erosive effect, by increasing the time which the drink is held in the mouth. Asking the patient to keep a diet diary is good practice for those for whom diet is suspected as being contributory to TSL.

Occasionally the cause cannot be identified. In this respect, the secretive nature of some eating disorders may be of relevance. Nevertheless, a caring approach may help patients to discuss their problems, possibly more readily with the dental nurse. The pattern of TSL in bulimic patients is well defined, with TSL typically affecting the palatal surfaces of the upper incisor, canine and possibly premolar teeth (fig. 4.13) and the occlusal surfaces of the mandibular molars and premolars. Amalgam restorations which are present in these teeth may appear 'proud' of the remaining tooth substance given that the amalgam is less soluble in gastric acids than tooth substance.

Abrasion may occasionally be identified as a cause of TSL, examples being the holding of a pipe stem between the teeth or pen chewing. It should also be noted that the abrasive action of toothbrushing is increased dramatically

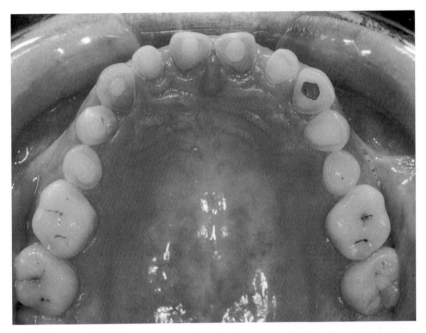

Figure 4.13 Tooth substance loss in a bulimic patient. (Reproduced by courtesy of George Warman Publications, Publishers of Dental update).

when it is carried out within 30 minutes of the teeth having been subjected to an erosive attack by citrus juices or food or by regurgitation of gastric acid.

While erosion has been considered to be the most prevalent reason for TSL, attrition, associated with clenching and/or grinding habits, is a cause of TSL in a proportion of patients. These patients may or may not be aware of their habits, but may complain of symptoms such as tender masticatory musculature on waking.

Potential causative factors of TSL should be identified, if possible, before referral. An assessment of the rapidity of progression is of value in assessing the need for referral and its urgency. As a general rule, increasing sensitivity of a tooth or group of teeth is an indication that wear is progressing faster than the deposition of reparative dentine. Also, chipping of incisal edges of anterior teeth is a sign that TSL is causing undermining of enamel at incisal edges. These may be reasons for patients to express anxiety and to request treatment.

6.8 EXAMINATION OF PATIENTS WITH TSL

A full clinical examination, to include radiographs, mounted study casts, intra-oral photographs and special investigations such as salivary tests should be carried out. Radiographs will provide an indication as to the amount of reparative dentine and the proximity of the pulp, in teeth affected by TSL, to the tooth surface. The radiographs may also show teeth in which damage from TSL has led to pulpal death and an associated area of periapical radiolucency. The tooth surfaces affected by TSL should be noted. For tooth wear to occur, teeth must, as a general rule, be well supported, but the clinician must not assume that all firm teeth are free from periodontal disease. A full periodontal assessment is therefore indicated. The vertical component of the occlusion should be assessed and the freeway space measured. Extraoral examination may reveal muscle hypertrophy, which may be as a result of bruxism, or enlarged parotid glands, which may be associated with bulimia.

Measurement of progression of TSL

Accurate measurement of progression of TSL is difficult, insofar that none of the methods commonly used are sufficiently accurate to detect small amounts of TSL. Study casts are the least expensive and most frequently used tool but these will only detect gross changes in tooth contour. Laser and computer scanning methods are available to the researcher, but at a cost which may preclude their use in general dental practice. There would therefore appear to be a need for the development of an accurate method of assessment of progression of tooth wear which is appropriate to general dental practice.

Prior to referral of a patient to a restorative specialist, the general dental practitioner should have:

- Taken a history in an effort to determine the possible causes of the patient's TSL
- Examined the patient to determine the severity of the TSL
- Made an assessment of the rate of progression of the disease

6.9 CLASSIFICATION OF TSL

TSL may be classified simply into:

    (i) localised and
    (ii) generalised.

(i) Rarely, large numbers of teeth are affected by TSL and TSL will be localised to a small number of teeth, usually in one arch. In general, when a small number of teeth are affected, these teeth alone should be treated. However, treatment should also include the determination of the cause of the TSL where possible so that the patient may be advised in respect of prevention of future TSL.

(ii) Generalised loss of tooth substance normally is as a result of several contributory factors, for example, the bruxist who also consumes excessive quantities of carbonated beverages, or, the bulimic who consumes excessive carbonated beverages and who brushes his/her teeth with an (abrasive) toothpaste shortly after vomiting. These patients will often require extensive restorative treatment, with the treatment dependent on the factors discussed below.

A widely accepted classification of the treatment of TSL was suggested by Tulloch and Watson in 1985. These clinicians classified their cases according to appearance and the need to increase the occlusal face height, as follows:

1. Appearance satisfactory
2. Appearance not satisfactory: No increase in occlusal face height required
3. Appearance not satisfactory: Increase in occlusal face height required
   (i) sufficient space available
   (ii) insufficient space available

For cases in category 1, treatment indicated is counselling, restoration of edentulous spaces where appropriate, treatment aimed at controlling any bruxist or clenching habits, adjustment and elimination of any occlusal interferences and routine dental treatment. For cases in category 2, treatment indicated is as for category 1 plus the treatment of the aesthetic problems by conventional restorative measures. Treatment of cases classified into Category 3 is more complex. It could be considered that patients in categories 1 and 2, and for whom the rate of progression of the TSL is low, are appropriate to treatment in general dental practice, although this is dependent on the experience, competence and confidence of the general dental practitioner.

6.10 COUNSELLING PATIENTS WITH TSL

In all cases, whether being referred or not, counselling the patient in respect of the possible cause of their TSL, practice-based treatment (of sensitivity, if present) and monitoring is appropriate. Patients should be counselled to return if sensitivity levels increase, or if enamel chips off anterior teeth, these being signs of progression of TSL. Patients should be appraised of the cause of their TSL and how further progress of TSL may be limited. For patients in whom the cause of the TSL is considered to be erosive, the following advice may be given: (Walmsley *et al.* 2002)

- reduce consumption of acidic drinks, such as carbonated beverages or citrus fruit drinks
- reduce the amount and frequency of intake
- avoid 'frothing' the drink
- avoid brushing the teeth for at least 30 minutes after drinking
- chill the drink – the erosive potential of cold drinks is less than warm drinks
- avoid drinking such drinks before bedtime or during the night

These patients should be informed that further TSL may occur unless the dietary advice listed above is adhered to.

For patients for whom the TSL is as a result of regurgitation of gastric acid, such as patients with gastric ulcers or hiatus hernia:

- The dentist and patient should collaborate with the patient's general medical practitioner in an effort to reduce oral effects caused by reflux of gastric acids
- The dentist should suggest that the patient minimises foods which cause regurgitation
- The use of an antacid mouthwash (e.g. bicarbonate of soda) immediately after regurgitation or vomiting should be suggested to neutralise the acid in the mouth.

Additionally, patients suffering from bulimia or anorexia may receive good help and advice from eating disorder self-help groups.

Other treatment of TSL is outwith the scope of this book. Readers are referred to a text on Restorative Dentistry, such as Restorative Dentistry by Walmsley and colleagues (2002).

6.11 CONCLUSION

A complete examination, and the making of a diagnosis/es, are essential prior to the referral of a patient. The majority of cases, other than those thought to be suffering from a tumour, are unlikely to require urgent referral. With regard to patients with TSL, only those patients suffering from rapidly progressing erosive TSL are likely to need urgent referral. Other forms of TSL progress only slowly (fig. 4.14). The general dental practitioner has an important role to play in the monitoring of patients, so that unnecessary referrals are minimised.

7.0 EVIDENCE-BASED DENTISTRY

History

In 1601, James Lancaster demonstrated that lemon juice was effective in the prevention of scurvy. The experiment was repeated in 1747 by James Lind with the same result. However, despite the frequent occurrence of scurvy on lengthy voyages, it was not until 1795 that the British Navy fully adopted the use of lemon juice and not until 1865 by the merchant marine (Haines and Jones 1994). So what caused the delay? The knowledge had been available for over a century, so the delay could not be caused by ignorance. Perhaps it was incompetence, but it appears that the delay occurred principally because the research findings were not disseminated to the potential users of the findings. The medical literature is littered with examples of research findings which have not been accepted in practice (Haines and Jones 1994). Recent examples include inadequate use of prophylactic anticoagulants for patients having orthopaedic surgery and inadequate treatment of children suffering from gastroenteritis (Guerrant and Bobak 1991, Laverick et al. 1991).

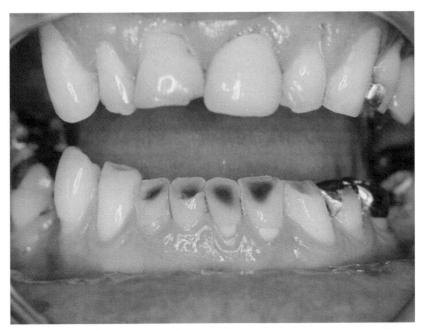

Figure 4.14 Patient referred urgently for assessment and treatment of TSL. However, at the consultation appointment, it become apparent that the patient's condition had not progressed for 20 years.

7.1 AN EVIDENCE-BASED APPROACH

Each time a dentist treats a patient, decisions are made which may relate to intangible factors with regard to that patient. General practitioners face daily uncertainty in clinical decision making and this uncertainty may often be concerned with intangible factors concerned with individual patients and in such cases it has been considered that the doctor's best resource may be his or her personal knowledge and intuition (Lancaster 1996). However, this uncertainty may be a result of incomplete knowledge, and in this respect, results of a recent study have indicated that clinicians have identified a need for more knowledge at the rate of two questions for every three patients who they examined (Covell *et al.* 1985). Finding the relevant knowledge is central to the 'evidence-based' approach to patient care. The concept of 'evidence-based' treatment involves the dissemination of results of clinical trials to the practitioner in primary dental care and encouraging the practitioner to look for and make sense of these results in order to apply it to everyday clinical decisions (Richards and Lawrence 1995).

Evidence may not only be the findings of published research but may include specific findings from a history and examination as detailed above. The research evidence will assist the clinician in deciding which interventions may be most effective while the clinical findings may harness clinical intuition from years of experience (Richards and Lawrence 1995). It is therefore essential that the decisions which are made for patients are made on a scientific basis, based on knowledge of what is the most appropriate treatment for a given situation. Increasingly, it is recognised that clinicians should be able to find the evidence which leads to correct treatment decisions, i.e. that they can carry out evidence-based treatment. This has been defined as the 'conscientious, explicit and judicious use of the current best evidence in making decisions about the care of individual patients' (Sackett *et al.* 1996). It also means the integration of individual clinical expertise with the best available evidence, with individual clinical evidence being the judgement that clinicians acquire through their clinical experience.

7.2 FINDING THE EVIDENCE

There are two sides to the evidence-based concept. First, the clinician must be able to find the appropriate knowledge, and then apply it. Four basic routes to finding good evidence have been suggested (fig. 4.15).

However, the research reports which could hold the answers are not always readily available to the dental practitioner, and moreover, there are around 500 journals related to dentistry. Evidence-based treatment is not restricted to randomised controlled trials and meta-analyses, but involves the tracking down of the most appropriate evidence. On an academic level, it may mean examination of the results of controlled clinical trials, and there are now organisations in place to collate and disseminate such information, for example, the Cochrane Centre in Oxford and the Cochrane Oral Health Group, based in Manchester. Ultimately, evidence-based dentistry will use

ROUTE	COMMENT
1. Ask someone!	Asking someone has the drawbacks that the expert consulted might not be up to date.
2. Consult a text book	Text books may be of value but they do not normally address specific questions.
3. Find a relevant article in your reprint file	Personal files are likely to be biased
4. Use a database such as MEDLINE	Arguably the quickest and simplest method of accessing evidence

Figure 4.15 Four routes to evidence (Richards and Lawrence 1995).

new technology to identify and retrieve information so that it will be available for those who wish to obtain it on a networked practice computer. By carrying out evidence-based treatment, the practitioner will be better able to cope with the demands of patients and improve the quality of their care. The hierarchy of evidence is shown in fig. 4.16.

Additionally, Goodman (1996) has suggested that prospective studies are preferred to retrospective ones, controlled studies are preferable to uncontrolled ones, randomised studies are preferable to non-randomised ones, blind studies in which patients (single-blind) or patients and investigators (double-blind) do not know who received what treatment are preferable to unblind ones and large studies preferable to small ones.

Neilson has provided an alternative to the above, with the level of evidence in decreasing order:
• Evidence obtained from at least one properly randomised controlled trial
• Evidence from well-designed controlled trials without randomisation
• Evidence from well-designed cohort or case control studies, preferably from more than one centre or research group
• Evidence from comparisons between times or places without an intervention
• Opinions of respected authorities based on clinical experience, or reports of expert committees.

Neilson (1995) noted that we traditionally depended most on the lowest level of evidence.

7.3 ARE LECTURERS ALWAYS EVIDENCE BASED?

The case has been described of the persuasive lecturer, who shows his/her audience a series of clinical slides illustrating the success of a technique, with the audience assuming that the technique would be successful in their hands, but some asking themselves whether they can question the validity of the

Meta analysis and systematic review
Large randomised controlled trial (Multi-centre)
Small randomised controlled trial (Single hospital/General Practice)
Case control study
Non-randomised trial with contemporaneous controls
Non-randomised trial with historical controls
Cross-sectional study
Series of consecutive cases
Individual case report

Figure 4.16 The hierarchy of evidence examining the effect of a clinical intervention, with the most rigorous being at the top after (Goodman 1996).

lecturer's findings. Lecturers should therefore be encouraged to state whether their findings are purely anecdotal or whether they have carried out a properly constructed scientific study, allowing them to draw firm conclusions from their findings. Lecturers may also experience a conflict of interest if much of their funding or sponsorship comes from one particular manufacturer.

7.4 A PROBLEM WITH EVIDENCE

While the evidence-based concept has served to place patient treatment on to a scientific basis rather than being based on anecdote, the evidence may take years to gather. The practice of dentistry on a totally evidence-based basis would therefore preclude the clinician from carrying out new forms of treatment on which the evidence has not been gathered. There may therefore be instances in which the clinician proceeds with a treatment which has no evidence for success, but which s/he may justify because data from laboratory experiments are promising, and/or because the treatment chosen is less invasive than the previously used alternatives for which evidence is available.

7.5 EVIDENCE: WHAT THE PATIENT REALLY WANTS TO KNOW

Patients, when discussing possible treatments, probably want to ask the following questions to their dentist, but generally don't!
• How good are you at the proposed treatment?

NUMBER ONE PATIENT QUESTION, never asked!
How good are you?
Additionally, patients will want to know
- Does it hurt?
- How much does it cost?
- How long will it last, i.e. is it cost effective?
- Does it last longer than alternatives?
- Is the treatment safe?

7.6 EVIDENCE NEEDS OF THE DENTIST

The evidence needs of the clinician are:
• As for patient
• Is the material or technique easy to use by clinician and nurse?
• Under what clinical situations is the material or technique best used?
• What are its clinical limitations?

On a practice basis, therefore, evidence-based dentistry should mean the setting up of the practice computer system to audit treatment performance and to determine the factors influencing success. In the current era of clinical governance, this is essential, but it is also appropriate so that patients may be in a position to make an informed decision regarding their own treatment. Some form of measurement of success is therefore essential. Methods of assessment of restorations used in research could be employed, but these are likely to be too rigorous for the purpose of informing patients, and may be too time consuming for a busy practice. A simplified system by which restorations may be assessed would therefore seem appropriate, for example a three-tier system where A=satisfactory, B=restoration present but some intervention needed, and C=restoration failure (Mike Busby, personal communication, 2002).

7.7 QUESTIONS FOR A SALES REPRESENTATIVE

A company sales representative may present a depth of knowledge about the materials produced by their company and its competitors, but it would seem reasonable to assume that they are unlikely to be able to present a totally unbiased viewpoint (Burke *et al.* 2002). Additionally, manufacturers of materials may also be under pressure from their marketing personnel to produce new claims for incorporation into advertising, or to reformulate a material in order to improve market position. It is for the clinician to ask the question whether s/he would prefer to purchase a material which performs well both clinically and in the research literature and which has not changed for a number of years (i.e. the manufacturer 'got it right' at the outset) or to purchase one which is altered minimally on a regular basis with claims such as increased fluoride content, or improved filler technology (i.e. the manufac-turer may not have 'got it right' at the outset, what guarantee is there that they have 'got it right' ever). Notwithstanding this, however, it has been considered that we should be grateful for the development of materials by manufacturers, because the market incentive has been the driving force to much that we use today.

It is therefore beholden to the clinician to ask questions which are perti-nent to the materials with which they are presented by a company represen-tative. Research in dental materials science is often laboratory based because of constraints of technology and control and this laboratory research may often be in the manufacturer's 'in house' laboratory rather than in the labora-tory of an independent organisation. It is necessary to verify, by laboratory research, that a given material is capable of withstanding the forces applied and functions required in the intraoral situation before that material is used on patients, either experimentally in the form of a trial or in the dental office under normal situations of payment. Principal advantages of laboratory research are the ability to control variables, produce comparative data between 'competing' and/or similar products, and to compare old with new. The difficulty comes in deciding whether any of the laboratory research may be applied appropriately to the clinical situation. Representatives should be able to substantiate the effectiveness of their materials by quoting independent research in the form of a properly structured research paper containing full details of the methods used, the results and their discussion and the conclusion(s). Such research should be published in a peer-reviewed journal, following which it will be in the public domain for further discussion.

Emling (1995) has considered that there are three levels of information (fig 4.17). It is for the reader to decide into which category the claims made in advertising or in meetings (and presented in fig 4.18) with sales representatives falls.

A number of claims taken from advertising material are presented in fig 4.18. Readers may like to place these claims into Emling's levels of information. From these it can be seen that claims appear to be made, often without any reference to the source of the claim, even if this is valid and available – i.e. there are few statements which could be considered to be at the optimum level III level of information.

Suggested questions for a dental sales representative therefore include (Burke *et al.* 2002):

General questions:

1. Is the evidence published in peer-reviewed journals?
2. Who supported the research – a company, the authors' institution, grant money, combination of these?

Level I information is that which is distilled into everyday language – 'It cleans better', 'it lasts longer', etc. This is the language that the majority of patients see and use in their everyday lives and it is beholden to the dental practitioner to be able to assess whether there is scientific validity to such claims by having a knowledge of the scientific literature.

Level II information may have a scientific basis, but the methodology and the full results are not in the public domain. Emling considers that this level of information is often that which appears in promotional material to back up a product, with a reference sometimes being given or the statement 'data on file' being made. The question should be asked, is this simply an opinion by a researcher, employee of the manufacturing company or a paid endorsement.

Level III information is the source itself – a research paper published in a peer-reviewed journal, with the standard sections of introduction/literature review, methods, results, discussion and conclusion.

Figure 4.17

(i) The all ceramic crown of choice!
Strongest all ceramic crown
Unsurpassed aesthetics
Easy preparation
Biocompatible (metal free)

(ii) The 'smart' restorative that's a real alternative to amalgam
Intelligent pH control releases active ions on demand, preventing or
significantly hampering the formation of secondary caries
Simple ultra-fast technique – up to 40% quicker to place than similar-sized
amalgam restorations

(iii) ** is a hybrid composite containing barium glass and fumed silica with a
submicron particle size, contains fluoride, is available in 8 Vita shades, can
be used for small restorations with difficult access, repairing margins...
This is a truly brilliant product.

(iv) One bond for all
Truly universal adhesive
Fluoride in the formulation provides fluoride to the tooth structure
Postoperative sensitivity is a problem of the past – a comprehensive study of
350 patients showed that when posterior composite restorations were placed
using this adhesive, no symptoms of sensitivity occurred. (Abstract reference
given.)
Bond strength at its peak
Elastomeric resins act as shock absorbers and help absorb setting
shrinkage

(v) Brilliant aesthetics and easy placement
Polishes to a natural brilliance
Extremely low water absorption to promote long term stability
Superior handling

(vi) Strength and aesthetics combined: Direct and Indirect restorations
Unique filler for maximum wear resistance and fracture toughness
Answers patient demands for a white filling – excellent polishability and
blends to tooth colour
Ease of use – non-sticky and non-slumping

(vii) no etch simplicity
greater strength and more clinical indications
more fluoride release

Figure 4.18 Statements made in a selection Advertisements.

Clinical trials:
1. Number of patients
2. Length of trials
3. Methodology (as in Table 4.1)

Safety studies
1. Number and type of animals
2. Type of test
3. If appropriate, does the material meet specification requirements?
4. Any other tests – cell culture, etc.

Adhesion/interfacial properties
1. Adhesion to enamel/dentine
2. How measured, tension, shear, other?
3. With or without thermal cycling?
4. When measured, one hour, one week?

Chemical properties
1. Solubility?
2. Swelling associated with absorption?
3. Release of fluoride – quantity, sustained release?

Setting properties
1. Shrinkage or expansion
2. Effect on bond strength
3. Working and setting time

Mechanical properties
1. Strength
2. Fracture toughness

Surface properties
1. Hardness
2. Abrasion resistance
3. Abrasion and wear of opposing tooth.
4. Surface roughness
5. Tendency for plaque accumulation

Aesthetic properties
1. Shades available
2. Potential for extrinsic staining
3. Potential for discolouration (intrinsic)

Practicability
1. Ease and time of placement
2. Cost
3. Cost of associated equipment (curing light, etc.).

In conclusion, it has been suggested that the ability to find and correctly interpret the information presented by advertisers and manufacturers is an integral aspect of 'evidence-based' clinical practice, given that blind acceptance of claims made by advertisers may lead to the disappointment of poor clinical performance (Burke *et al.* 2002). It is therefore beholden to manufacturers to substantiate claims made in advertising and for researchers to present their data in a manner which can be readily understood by the clinician. In turn, it is essential that the researcher has used the correct methodology and that, where possible, the publisher of research has ensured the validity of the publication. However, in the final analysis it is important that the clinician has the ability to scientifically appraise the data with which s/he is presented, and it may be considered that this ability will become more important as patients increasingly request evidence as to the potential success and cost-effectiveness of their treatment options.

8.0 CLINICAL GOVERNANCE

The concept of clinical governance was introduced in the 1990s in the wake of a number of episodes in which incompetence by medical staff had, at best, gone un-noticed or, at worst, had been noticed but not been acted upon, principally because figures for success rates in different units, or even by different surgeons in the same unit, were not compared.

Dentists do not generally deal with matters of life and death in the way that medical practitioners, physicians and surgeons do, but it is nevertheless essential that the treatments carried out by a dentist are subjected to the principles of clinical governance.

There are several strands to this:
- Results should be compared against a standard
- Variations from this standard should be investigated
- Improvements should be identified and implemented: this then becomes the new standard against which comparisons are made
- A commitment to lifelong learning and continuing professional development

Clinical governance is associated with doing all that is necessary to maximise quality. However, to do this, it is essential that a means of measuring quality is available. This could take the form of measuring the oral health of patients in the practice using, for example, an Index of Oral Health (see Chapter 2 Section 1.8) or developing a method for auditing the success of different types of restoration. It could also take the form of an assessment of the incidence of adverse occurrences, such as post-operative pain following root canal therapy. The importance of developing systems for computerised recording of such information becomes obvious when the concepts of clinical governance are considered. It is also essential that sufficient clinical information is recorded in patient records, so that its analysis is possible. The addition of another strand to the list above may therefore be appropriate, namely, the keeping of full, contemporaneous records of patient treatment.

The concept of lifelong learning is also central to clinical governance, as it is essential that the clinician keeps abreast of current information. While it is tempting for the clinician to undertake postgraduate education in the areas of his/her greatest interest, each dentist should analyse the deficiencies in his/her knowledge and update these areas by way of courses, e-learning and reading.

REFERENCES

Anusavice KJ. Treatment regimens in preventive and restorative dentistry. *J Am Dent Assoc* 1995(6);126:727–40.

Anusavice KJ. Efficacy of nonsurgical management of the initial caries lesion. *J Dent Educ* 1997;61:895–905.

Arnold C, Brookes V, Griffiths J, Maddock S, Theophilou S. (2000) Guidelines for oral health care for people with a physical disability. Report of BSDH Working Group. UK. British Society for Disability and Oral Health.

Balshi TJ. Sequential treatment planning. *Gen Dent* 1980;28:113–17.

Barbakow F, Gaberthuel T, Lutz F, Schuepbach P. Maintenance of amalgam restorations. *Quintessence Int* 1988;19:861–70.

Barbotte E, Guillemin F, Chai N, *et al.* (2001). *Prevalence of impairments, disabilities, handicaps and quality of life in the general population: a review of the literature.* Bulletin of the World Health Organization; 79:1047–55.

Blinkhorn AS. (1993) Evaluation and planning of oral health promotion programmes. In (ed. L. Schou and AS. Blinkhorn) *Oral health promotion.* Oxford: Oxford Medical Publications.

Brook PH, Shaw WC. The development of orthodontic treatment priority index. *European Journal of Orthodontics* 1989;11:309–20.

Brown JP. Indicators for caries management from the patient history. *J Dent Educ* 1997; 61:855–60.

Burke FJT, McHugh S, MacPherson L, Hosey M-T, Shaw L, Delargy S., Dopheide B. UK dental practitioners understanding of ART. PEF IADR abstract No 224.

Burke FJT, McCord JF, Cheung SW. The provision of emergency dental care by general dental practitioners in an urban area. *Dent Update* 1994;21:184–6.

Burke FJT, McCord JF, Hoad-Reddick G, Cheung SW. (DfES 1995) Provision of domiciliary dental care in a UK urban area: results of a survey. *Primary Dental Care* 2: 47–50.

Burke FJT, Wilson NHF. Measuring oral health: an historical view and details of a contemporary oral health index (OHX). *Int Dent J* 1995;45:358–70.

Burke FJT, Qualtrough AJE, Hale RW. Dentin-bonded all-ceramic crowns: Current Status. *J Am Dent Assoc* 1998;129:455–60.

Burke FJT, Goodall CA, Hayes F. Appropriate and inappropriate referrals to a unit of conservative dentistry. *Primary Dental Care* 1999;6:141–4.

Burke FJT, Shortall ACC, Combe EC, Aitchison TC. Assessing restorative dental materials 2: questions for a sales representative. *Dent Update* 2002;29:244–8.

Cohen LK. Converting unmet need for care to effective demand. *International Dental Journal* 1987;37:114–16.

Covell DG, Uman GC, Manning PR. Information needs in office practice: are they being met? *Ann Intern Med* 1985;103:596–9.

de St. Georges J. The emergency patient. *Br Dent J* 1990;169:37–8.

DfES. (DfES 1995) Disability Discrimination Act 1995. Code of practice, rights of access, goods, facilities, services and premises. London. Department for Education and Skills Publication Number DLE9.

DH (2002). *NHS dentistry: options for change*. London: Department of Health.

Edwards DM, Merry AJ. Disability Part 2: access to dental services for disabled people. A questionnaires survey of dental practices in Merseyside. *British Dental Journal* 2002; 193:253–5.

Ekstrand K, Qvist V, Thylstrup A. Light microscope study of the effect of probing in occlusal surfaces. *Caries Res* 1987;21:368–74.

Emling RC. Understanding laboratory and clinical research: an overview. *J Clin Dent* 1995;VI:157–60.

Espelid I, Tveit AB. Diagnosis of secondary caries and crevices adjacent to amalgam. *Int Dent J* 1991;41:359–64.

European Commission. Report and recommendations concerning clinical proficiencies required for the practice of dentistry in the European Union.

European Society of Endodontology. Consensus report of the European Society of Endodontology on quality guidelines for endodontic treatment. *Int Endod J* 1994; 27:115–24.

Evans R, Shaw WC. Preliminary evaluation of an illustrated scale for rating dental attractiveness. *European Journal of Orthodontics* 1987;9:314–18.

Fisher FJ. Toothache and cracked cusps. *Br Dent J* 1982;153:298–300.

Fiske J, Lewis D. (2000) The development of standards for domiciliary dental care services: guidelines and recommendations. Report of BSDH Working Group. UK. British Society for Disability and Oral Health.

Fox NA, Thompson R. Audit of new patient referrals. *Orthodontic Audit Working Party Newsletter RCS Eng* 1993;5:6–7.

Freeman R, Adams EK, Gelbier S. The provision of primary dental care for patients with special needs. *Primary Dental Care* 1997;4:31–4.

Freeman R. Social exclusion, barriers and accessing dental care: thoughts on planning responsive dental services. *Brazilian Journal of Oral Sciences* 2002;1:34–37.

Frencken J, Phantumvanit P, Pilot T, Songpaisan Y, van Amerongen E. Manual for Atraumatic Restorative treatment. 1997, WHO Collaboarting Centre for Oral Health Services research, Groningen.

Gibson BJ, Freeman R. Dangerousness and dentistry: an explanation of dentists' reactions and responses to the treatment of HIV-seropositive patients. *Community Dentistry and Oral Epidemiology* 1996a;24:341–5.

Gibson BJ, Freeman R. Dentists practising in Lothian treat HIV-seropositive patients: is this a resolution of conflict or a case of Hobson's choice? *British Dental Journal* 1996b; 180:34–7.

Goodman C. Literature searching and evidence interpretation for assessing health care practices. 1996, Stockholm, The Swedish Council on Technology Assessment in Health Care.

Griffiths J, Jones V, Leeman I., *et al.* (2000) *Oral health care for people with mental health problems: guidelines and recommendations*. Report of BSDH Working Group. UK. British Society for Disability and Oral Health.

Guerrant RI, Bobak DA. Bacterial and protozoal gastroenteritis. *N Engl J Med* 1991; 325:327–40.

Guide for dental students and practitioners. Medical Defence Union, Dental Division. London, 1992.

Haines A, Jones R. Implementing findings of research. *Br Med J* 1994;308:1488–92.

Hall WB, Roberts WE, LaBarre EE. Decision Making in Dental Treatment Planning. 1994, Mosby Year Book, St.Louis, Missouri 63146, US.

Hartnett AC, Shiloah J. The treatment of acute necrotising ulcerative gingivitis. *Quintessence Int* 1991;22:95–100.

Jinks GM. Fluoride-impregnated cements and their effect on the activity of interproximal caries. *J Dent Child* 1963;30:87–92.

Kay EJ, Locker D. Is dental health education effective? *Community Dentistry and Oral Epidemiology* 1996;24:231–5.

Kayser AF, Battistuzzi PGFCM, Snoek PA, Plasmans PJ, Spanauf AJ. The implementation of a problem-oriented treatment plan. *Aust Dent J* 1988;33:18–22.

Kayser AF, Witter DJ, Spanauf AJ. Overtreatment with removable partial dentures in shortened dental arches. *Aust Dent J* 1987;32:178–82.

Kidd EAM. The diagnosis and management of the 'early' carious lesion in permanent teeth. *Dent Update* 1984;11:69–80.

Kidd EAM. Caries diagnosis within restored teeth. In Anusavice KJ (ed) Quality evaluation of dental restorations. p. 111, Chicago, Quintessence Publishing Co., 1989.

Kidd EAM, Smith BGN. Pickard's Manual of operative dentistry. Oxford: Oxford University Press, 1990.

Kidd EAM, Toffenetti F, Mjor IA. Secondary caries. *Int Dent J* 1992;42:127–38.

Kirschen R. Orthodontic clinical screening in under a minute. *British Dental Journal* 1998;185:224–6.

Lancaster T. What is evidence-based medicine? Update. 1May 1996:434–5.

Laverick MD, Croal SA, Mollan RAB. Orthopaedic surgeons and thromboprophylaxis. *Br Med J* 1991;303:549–50.

Levine, RS.(1996) *The scientific basis of dental health education. a policy document.* 4th edition. London: Health Education Authority.

Mabelya L, Freeman R. Application of the primary health care approach to oral health systems in underdeveloped countries. *Odontstomal Trop* 1985;VIII:147–253

Maintaining Standards: what the patient expects. General Dental Council, London, 2000.

McKeown T. (1979) *The role of medicine. Dream, mirage or nemesis?* Oxford: Blackwell.

Merry AJ, Edwards DM. Disability Part 1: the Disability Discrimination Act (DfES 1995) – implications for dentists. *British Dental Journal* 2002;193:199–201.

Mjor IA. Amalgam and composite restorations: longevity and reasons for replacement. In ed., Anusavice K. Quality Evaluation of Dental Restorations. Chicago, Quintessence Publishing Co., 1989, pp. 61–8.

Mjor IA. Glass ionomer cement restorations and secondary caries: a preliminary report. *Quintessence Int* 1996;27:171–4.

Mjor IA, Gordan VV. A review of atraumatic restorative treatment (ART). *Int Dent J* 1999;49:127–31.

Naasan MA, Watson TF. Conventional glass ionomers as posterior restorations. A status report for the American Journal of Dentistry. *Am J Dent* 1998;11:36–45.

Nehammer CF. Treatment of the emergency patient. *Br Dent J* 1985;158:245–53.

Neilson P. It works in my hands. Why isn't that enough. *Quintessence Int* 1998;29:799–802.

Nunn J. (2000) Disability – a Context. In (ed. J. Nunn) *Disability and Oral Health.* London: FDI World Dental Press Ltd.

O'Brien K, McComb JL, Fox N, Bearn D, Wright J. Do dentists refer orthodontic patients inappropriately? *British Dental Journal* 1996;181:132–6.

Oliver CH, Nunn JH. The accessibility of dental treatment to adults with physical disabilities in northeast England. *Spec Care Dentist* 1996;16:204–9.

Pienihakkinen K. Caries prediction through combined use of incipient caries lesions, salivary buffering capacity, lactobacilli and yeasts in Finland. *Community Dent. Oral Epidemiol* 1987;15:325–30.

Prochanska JO, DiClemente CC. Stages and processes of self change of smoking: toward an integrative model of change. *Journal of Consulting and Clinical Psychology* 1983; 5:390–5.

Randall R, Wilson NHF. Glass ionomers: systematic review of a secondary caries treatment effect. *J Dent Res* 1997;76:1066 (Abstract 378).

Report of the Advisory Committee on the training of dental practitioners XV/E/8316/8/93 Brussels, 1993.

Richards D, Lawrence A. Evidence based dentistry. *Br Dent J* 1995;179:270–3.

Richardson A. Interceptive Orthodontics 4 edn. 1999 BDJ Books London ISBN0 904588 56 4.

Rollnick S, Mason P, Butler C. (2000) *Health Behaviors Change: A Guide for Practitioners.* London: Churchill Livingstone.

Rosenstock IM. What research in motivation suggest for public health. *American Journal of Public Health* 1960;50:295–301.

Royal College of Surgeons Clinical (2001) *Clinical Guidelines and Integrated Care Pathways for the Oral Health Care of People with Learning Disabilities.* London: Royal College of Surgeons.

Sackett DL, Rosenberg WMC, Gray JAM, Haynes RB, Richardson WS. Evidence based medicine: what it is and what it isn't. *Br Med J* 1996;312:71–2.

Shillingburg HT, Hobo SH. Fundamentals of Fixed Prosthodontics, 3rd edn. Quintessence Publishing Co., Chicago, 1997.

Simonsen RJ. Preventive resin restorations: three year results. *J Am Dent Assoc* 1980; 100:535–9.

Smith M, Freeman R. (2003) Do health care professionals refer housebound people to dental services? Referral behaviours and characteristic factors. *Journal of Disability and Oral Health* 2003;4:51–57.

Suddick RP, Dodds MWJ. Caries activity estimates and implications: insights into risk versus activity. *J Dent Educ* 1997;61:876–83.

The Dental Contract: detailed guidance. Department of Health and Social Services. October 1990.

Tveit AB, Espelid I. Class II amalgams: interobserver variations in replacement decisions and diagnosis of caries and crevices. *Int Dent J* 1992;42:12–18.

Verdonschot M. Dental treatment planning + problem solving. PhD Thesis, 1984, Katholieke Universitieit of Nijmegen.

Walmsley AD, Walsh TF, Burke FJT, Shortall ACC, Lumley PJ, Hayes-Hall R. Restorative Dentistry 2002, Churchill-Livingstone, Edinburgh.

Watson ML, Burke FJT. Investigation and treatment of patients affected by tooth substance loss: a review. *Dent Update* 2000;27:1175–83.

Watson IB, Tulloch EN. Clinical assessment of cases of tooth surface loss. *Br Dent J* 1985;159:144–8.

Wilson NHF, Burke FJT, Mjor IA. Reasons for placement and replacement of restorations of direct restorative materials by a selected group of practitioners in the United Kingdom. *Quintessence Int* 1997;28:245–8.

World Health Organisation (1978). UNICEF Primary health care, Alma Ata 1978. 'Health For All' Series No 10. Geneva: World Health Organisation

World Health Organisation (1986) *The Ottawa Charter for Health Promotion.* Ontario: WHO.

World Health Organisation (1981) *Global Strategy for Health for all by the Year 2000.* Geneva. WHO.

Young practitioners guide to Orthodontics. British Orthodontic Society 1996.

5 Essential business principles of dental practice

5.1 ESSENTIAL ACCOUNTING AND INSURANCE (MIKE GRACE)

Essential accounting

Understanding accounts is an essential part of both preparing for and running any business, including a dental practice. This applies to both practice owners and associates, as a good financial understanding is required for organising your own personal accounts as well.

For the purposes of running a business there are a number of financial models which are essential to effective financial management of that business (outlined below).

Financial models used in running a business

- Net Worth
- Profit and Loss
- Balance Sheet

- Budgeting
- Cash Flow Forecast

Two of these, the balance sheet and the profit and loss accounts, are traditionally prepared by an accountant for the purpose of taxation, and thus known as the 'accounts'. The others (cash flow forecast and budget) are useful in the management of the business but are not required by the Inland Revenue. Because they are not legally required, this often means the business owner does not prepare them, which is a pity as they can be both useful and valuable documents.

The three basic questions

The most basic financial questions you need to be able to answer are:
- Where are we now?
- How have we been doing so far?
- What do we think will happen in the future?

These can be broken down further into:
- How much money does the business have and where is it?
- Is the money in the business shrinking or growing?
- What is my financial plan for money coming into the business and going out of the business over the next 12 months (or so)?

The answers to the first two questions can be found by looking at the balance sheet and the profit and loss accounts (P&L) as described in fig. 5.1.

The third question is answered by a financial budget and a cash flow forecast.

The balance sheet

Most businesses need finance to get started. The balance sheet will tell you how much money was required to get the business going, where it came

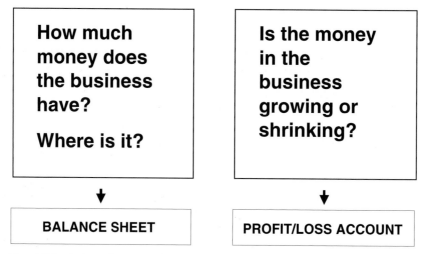

Figure 5.1 The basic functions of the balance sheet and profit and loss accounts. Reproduced with permission from the BDJ book "Finance For The Terrified".

from, and what it has been spent on. Thus, the balance sheet is a document that explains how much the business is worth at the time, taking into account all the years it has operated. It is usually described as a snapshot of the business on the day it was drawn up. This means a balance sheet could change quite substantially depending on the day, which is worth considering if you are looking at a balance sheet when deciding whether to purchase a practice or not. For example the balance sheet of a practice that purchased a substantial amount of new equipment (refurbishing the entire practice for example) would look quite different on the day after the purchase than on the day before.

In its simplest form the balance sheet looks like fig. 5.2.

On the left side we can see how much money is invested into the practice and where that money has come from (the owner's original money – called share capital) and some long-term loans (called loan capital) plus profits retained after the owner has drawn out the amount s/he wishes to live on. On the right side we can see how that money has been spent (the assets are things the practice owns). Please note that the amounts are unrealistic and purely to show the principles involved.

Obviously the amount of money invested into the business (the left side of fig. 5.2) and the explanation of how the money has been spent (the right side of fig 5.2) should be the same, or in other words it should 'balance', hence the name 'balance sheet'.

Balance sheets can often look different because of the way that accountants choose to draw them up. The simplest structure is like the one illustrated in fig. 5.3A – showing a balance between the capital, liabilities and profit and the actual assets of the business. This type of balance sheet balances where the money is now (the assets) with where it came from (capital plus liabilities) plus what you have earned (profit).

Where the money came from		Where the money is now	
SHARE CAPITAL		**FIXED ASSETS**	
Savings	5000	Premises	50 000
		Equipment	10 000
LOAN CAPITAL		Fixtures/fittings	2000
Mortgage	50 000		
HP on equipment	10 000	**CURRENT ASSETS**	
		Stock	2000
Profit	1000	Cash	2000
Total	66 000	**Total**	66 000

Figure 5.2 An example balance sheet illustrating where the money came from and where it is now. Reproduced from the BDJ book "Finance For The Terrified".

A

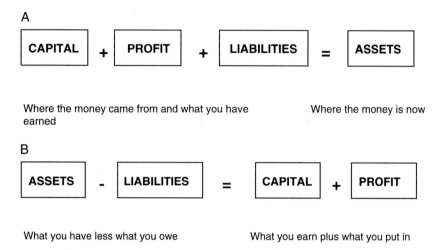

| CAPITAL | + | PROFIT | + | LIABILITIES | = | ASSETS |

Where the money came from and what you have earned

Where the money is now

B

| ASSETS | - | LIABILITIES | = | CAPITAL | + | PROFIT |

What you have less what you owe

What you earn plus what you put in

Figure 5.3 A: The traditional formula for a balance sheet. B: The more common formula for a balance sheet. Reproduced with permission from the BDA book "Finance For The Terrified".

However, most accountants prefer the format shown in fig. 5.3B, which balances what money you have (assets) less the money you owe (liabilities) with what you put into the business (capital), plus what you have earned (profit). The term capital account is often used to describe the capital and profit, and represents what would be left if the owners sold all their assets and paid off their liabilities. In other words, it represents what the owners have got in the business in financial terms.

Thus a more usual format for a balance sheet is Table 5.1 which represents the same amounts as in fig. 5.2, but written differently. You will note all the amounts are the same, but the final balance (£6000) is different because of the way the accountant has written it. However, it still balances.

Thus the value of the balance sheet is that it shows how much money is currently in the business, and how that money has been acquired and spent.

Profit and loss accounts

The profit and loss account (P&L) shows how much money has come into the practice (income) and how much has been spent (expenditure) in the current period (usually a maximum of a year). The profit is the extra money the business has made (in other words, the excess of money taken in sales over money spent in operating the business). Table 5.2 shows a basic P&L (again with token amounts to show the principle).

The P&L only shows money spent on running the business, so it does not show the cost of purchase of any capital expenditure (money spent on buying

Table 5.1 The general structure of a balance sheet as presented by most accountants

Assets	
Bank account	2000
Premises	50 000
Equipment	10 000
Fixtures/fittings	2000
Stock	2000
	66 000
Liabilities	
Mortgage	(50 000)
HP	(10 000)
	(60 000)
Total net assets	6000
Financed by:	
Capital Accounts	
Smith	3000
Jones	3000
	6000

Table 5.2 The general structure of a profit and loss model

Income	70 000
Expenses	
Materials	10 000
Laboratory fees	7000
Wages	12 500
Services	3000
Rates	2000
Other	3000
Loan interest	2000
Bank charges	1000
Accountant	3000
Depreciation	1000
Insurance	500
Total	45 000
Profit	25 000

Tables 5.1 and 5.2: Reproduced with permission from the BDJ book "Finance For The Terrified".

equipment and other major capital purchases) but will include any interest or fees paid on loan capital and share capital (as these are part of running the business).

Apart from the first year in any business the P&L usually compares the current year with the previous year. Table 5.3 illustrates this, and we can draw some interesting conclusions from the data. First, profit is down compared with the previous year (£33 084 compared with £40 537). The main reason for this would appear to be the fact that income has hardly risen, but expenses have. There may be an adequate explanation for this (the owner of the practice may have reduced the time spent in the practice by taking up a position somewhere else, such as in another practice or a part-time position in a local hospital), but if there is no obvious reason then the reducing profit would be an area of concern.

If we did not have the actual figures for both years on the same paper then this loss of profit might not be so obvious (although a good accountant would draw your attention to it). This layout also makes it easier to compare figures between years to see where costs have risen.

The P&L is an easy model to understand, but far more value comes from considering the P&L if appropriate action is taken. However, as the P&L tends to be produced several months after the end of the financial year it could be rather late to discover some of these financial items, which is why you should be aware of increasing costs and decreasing income as soon as it happens. For this a budget is an ideal financial model.

Budgets

Budgets are simply financial models that look at what we think is going to happen financially in the future and then compares it on a monthly basis to see what actually does happen.

Thus a budget tries to predict both income and expenditure (normally for a 12-month period although you can have a budget for any period of time) first, then compares the prediction with the reality, and then acts as a guide as to how to react.

For example, Table 5.4 shows a typical budget approximately halfway through a 12-month period. The three columns marked 'Current period' refer to the month just finished, while the column marked 'Year to date' refers to the budget compared with actual from the start of the financial year to the end of the month just completed. Say your financial year ran from January 1st to December 31st, then at the end of June the budget might well look like Table 5.4.

Taking the 'Current period' column first, we can see that we assumed income would be £8300 and expenditure would be £3610. This would have been estimated first taking into account the previous year's figures plus an allowance for inflation plus any other influences (such as the addition of an

Table 5.3 A sample profit and loss account

A.N Dentist, BDS
Profit and Loss Account
Year ended December 1996

	2000/2001		1999/2000	
Gross fees	173 474		172 271	
Less associates remuneration	57 191		54 577	
Net fees	116 283		117 694	
Less expenses				
Direct expenses				
Materials and drugs	13 478		11 004	
Wages and salaries	27 348		25 507	
Laboratory expenses	18 854		16 692	
Course fees	540		200	
	60 220	60 220	53 403	53 403
Establishment expenses				
Rent	8302		8302	
Rates	700		650	
Light and heat	1032		984	
Repairs and maintenance	146		102	
Insurance	733		620	
	10 913	10 913	10 658	10 658
General expenses				
Motor and travelling	2503		2850	
Telephone	1080		926	
Printing, postage	932		703	
Stationary	642		496	
Accountancy fees	1450		1380	
Sundry expenses	1143		742	
	7750	7750	7097	7097
Financial expenses				
Bank charges & interest	2503		2846	
Loan interest (equipment)	890		1040	
Hire purchase (car)	1662		1662	
Bad debts	1342		1586	
	6397	6397	7134	7134
Depreciation				
Fixtures and equipment	2560		2560	
Motor vehicle	3109		3582	
	5669	5669	6142	6142
Total overheads		83 199		77 337
Net profit for year		33 084		40 357

Reproduced with permission from the BDJ book "Finance For The Terrified".

Table 5.4 A model of a budget approximately 6 months through the year

	Current period			Year to date		
	(budget)	(actual)	Variance	(budget)	(actual)	Variance
Income						
Fees	£8000	£8744	£744	£65 000	£69 345	£4345
Other	£300	£300	£0	£1200	£753	£447
Total income	£8300	£9044	£744	£66 200	£70 098	£3898
Fixed expenses						
Rent & Business Rates	£400	£400	£0	£2000	£2377	£377
Heat & Light	£270	£299	£29	£900	£860	(£40)
Repairs		£54	£54	£600	£366	(£234)
Other	£100	£26	(£74)	£600	£844	£244
Loans	£100	£100	£0	£1000	£1000	£0
Total fixed	£870	£879	£9	£5100	£5447	£347
Running expenses						
Wages	£1600	£1600	£0	£18 000	£17 560	(£440)
Laboratory Fees	£800	£647	(£153)	£12 000	£8930	(£3070)
Materials	£250	£230	(£20)	£2000	£2680	£680
Bank Interest	£50	£76	£26	£1000	£1600	£600
Postage	£40	£26	(£14)	£300	£580	£280
Total running	£2740	£2579	(£161)	£33 300	£31 350	(£1950)
Total expenses	£3610	£3458	(£152)	£38 400	£36 797	(£1603)
Profit/Loss	£4690	£5586	£896	£27 800	£33 301	£5501

Reproduced with permission from the BDJ book "Finance For The Terrified".

extra dentist or a full-time dentist switching to part-time). The actual income and expenditure (middle column in the 'Current period' column) is £9044 and £3458. This has resulted in a variance overall of £896 more profit than we budgeted for.

If we now look at the 'Year to date' column we can see that comparing the budget with the actual shows a healthy trend of earning more and spending less than our budget (by £5501). Thus the ability to know how well we are doing compared with budget enables us to plan more confidently as well as spot when things are going wrong sooner and take appropriate action.

Cash flow forecast

The final model is the cash flow forecast. This model (which always looks far more complex than it is) estimates how cash will flow into and out of the bank account. The principle of estimating the figures is the same as estimating a budget, but now we look at the money going through the bank account and see when we are going to need an overdraft facility as well as when we will have surplus money that it might be sensible to move to a high-interest account.

Table 5.5 shows a completed cash flow forecast (again the figures are not meant to be realistic). On the top left (in the row marked b/f which stands for 'brought forward') there is an overdraft of £4000. Under income we have estimated the income, with some variations for seasonal earnings and holidays. Remember this is the actual cash paid into the bank, not the money when it is earned, which can be quite different in timing depending on when you collect money and when you are paid. The expenses figures also relate to when the money is paid out.

In this model, the drawings and money allowed for tax have also been included (as this also comes from the same bank account). The figure in the row marked 'balance' is the actual amount in the bank on the last day of the month, and this figure is carried forward to the b/f row at the top of the next month.

In this case the cash flow forecast predicts that the overdraft will be no longer necessary after May, apart from a slight dip in September. This kind of information is helpful for the bank, and reassuring for you. Although the actual amounts will not be the same as your initial analysis, by recording the actual figures as they occur you will see fluctuations in cash flow and be able to predict appropriate action depending on what happens.

Finding a good accountant

Finding a good accountant is much the same as finding any professional adviser, be it a doctor, dentist or solicitor. The key is to find the right person for you, and ensure that s/he takes account of your wishes and feelings as well as being able to do the job.

Table 5.5 A model of a cash flow forecast

Cash Flow Forecast

	Jan	Feb	Mar	Apr	May	Jun	Jul	Aug	Sep	Oct	Nov	Dec
Balance b/f	(£4000)	(£3310)	(£3475)	(£4525)	(£2835)	£0	£3190	£6490	£625	(£415)	£1975	£3,210
Income												
Fees	£8000	£7000	£7000	£9000	£10000	£11000	£11000	£3000	£7000	£10000	£9000	£8000
Other	£300	£300	£300	£300	£300	£300	£300	£300	£300	£300	£300	£300
Total income	£8300	£7300	£7300	£9300	£10300	£11300	£11300	£3300	£7300	£10300	£9300	£8300
Fixed expenses												
Rent & Business Rates	£400	£400	£400	£400	£400	£400	£400	£400	£400	£400	£400	£400
Heat & Light	£270		£300	£270		£300	£270		£300	£270		£300
Repairs		£125			£125			£125			£125	
Insurance			£380				£90				£300	
Total fixed	£670	£525	£1080	£670	£525	£700	£760	£525	£700	£670	£825	£700
Running expenses												
Wages	£1,600	£1,600	£1,600	£1,600	£1,600	£1,600	£1,900	£1,900	£1,900	£1,900	£1,900	£1,900
Laboratory Fees	£800	£800	£800	£800	£800	£800	£800	£800	£800	£800	£800	£800
Materials	£250	£250	£250	£250	£250	£250	£250	£250	£250	£250	£250	£250
Bank Interest	£50	£50	£50	£50	£50	£50	£50	£50	£50	£50	£50	£50
Postage	£40	£40	£40	£40	£40	£40	£40	£40	£40	£40	£40	£40
Telephone			£330			£470			£400			£480
Accountant								£1400				
Other	£100	£100	£100	£100	£100	£100	£100	£100	£100	£100	£100	£100
Loans	£100	£100	£100	£100	£100	£100	£100	£100	£100	£100	£100	£100
Total running	£2940	£2940	£3270	£2940	£2940	£3410	£3240	£4640	£3640	£3240	£3240	£3720
Total Expenses	£3610	£3465	£4350	£3610	£3465	£4110	£4000	£5165	£4340	£3910	£4065	£4420
Profit/Loss	£4690	£3835	£2950	£5690	£6835	£7190	£7300	(£1865)	£2960	£6390	£5235	£3880
Drawings	£3000	£3000	£3000	£3000	£3000	£3000	£3000	£3000	£3000	£3000	£3000	£3000
Income tax	£1000	£1000	£1000	£1000	£1000	£1000	£1000	£1000	£1000	£1000	£1000	£1000
Balance	(£3310)	(£3475)	(£4525)	(£2835)	£0	£3190	£6490	£625	(£415)	£1975	£3210	£3090

Reproduced with permission from the BDJ book "Finance For The Terrified".

When looking for an accountant, whilst personal recommendation is helpful, remember that what different people want from an adviser differs, and what other people expect and want from their accountant may not be the same as you would want.

It is always sensible to visit several possible accountants to get a feeling of what they are like and how well they deal with you. Beware the 'expert' who will try and blind you with jargon, or the accountant who wants a client to simply sign on the dotted line when required. If a professional starts an interview by asking you what you want (instead of telling you what he or she can do for you) then you are on the right track.

Before the visit work out what you actually want. Do you want an accountant who will do all your accounts (including your cash flow, budgets, bank account details, etc.)? If you do you will pay a lot more, but it may be what you want. Do you want an accountant who will discuss future objectives, advise on your financial strategy, and act as a personal financial adviser? Do you want an accountant who will simply deal with your tax affairs? Whatever it is, make sure you know before you visit.

When you visit (and make sure you visit them first) look at the premises and the impression this creates. Make notes during the visit (you will not be able to remember later) and ask all the questions you need to. Be sure to ask about fees, and how they are calculated. Some accountants charge by the hour, some work on a fixed fee basis (unless something special comes up) and some work on commission. Never be afraid to ask about fees, and beware if you do not get a straight answer. After all, you are paying.

Finally, once you have made your choice, never be afraid to change if you are not happy. It may be awkward, but working with an accountant you do not like, do not understand or cannot trust is financial suicide.

Initial insurance requirements

There are two basic forms of insurance, personal (such as life insurance) and non-personal (such as motor insurance and household insurance). I shall only be dealing with one form of non-personal insurance, a practice expenses policy, and two forms of personal insurance (life and permanent health).

The purpose of personal insurance is to protect your income in the event of three main life situations:
- death
- permanent disability
- retirement (which usually involves a form of insurance known as a pension)

Thus individuals who have some way of protecting their income in any of the above situations (such as a substantial inheritance, alternative funds, assets to sell, etc.) may not need insurance, but for most people some form of personal insurance is usually advisable.

Life insurance

Life insurance has two main functions built into each policy, a protection element and an investment element. Different policies focus on one or other of these two main functions. In the past the policies could be broadly divided into three main types, depending on their emphasis on either protection or investment:

Term assurance: This is purely a form of protection for a fixed term. If you do not die before the term is completed then you receive nothing in return, which is why this type of policy is the cheapest.

Whole life: This policy lasts until you die (if you want it to) and part of each premium is invested, so you can 'cash in' the policy before you die. However the investment element of a 'whole of life' is fairly small, making this a poor form of investment. The advantage of this policy is that the company cannot cancel it should you develop a medical condition later in life.

Investment or savings: This type of policy simply uses a minimal life insurance function to provide tax benefits for saving money. These policies were very popular for 'school fees' schemes allowing people to save a regular monthly amount and have the money available at annual stages to help fund school fees. These days their value is limited because the tax benefits are now very limited (if at all) and there are many other options available to save with tax advantages.

The thing to remember with life insurance is that protection of income in the event of death should be the main reason for acquiring a policy. As the person taking out the policy will be dead, the only point of having life insurance is to protect dependents who rely on your income (such as a spouse and children) or to pay off a mortgage. If you have no mortgage and your dependents have their own income to rely on (or you have no dependents) then there is no real need to have life insurance. The only reason for having a policy before it is needed would be to protect your income should you develop a health condition later making you uninsurable or to start a policy early because it is cheaper the younger you are. However the cost of the 'unnecessary' premiums would need to be balanced against the higher costs of starting a policy later (probably a fairly minimal increase).

Permanent Health Insurance (PHI)

This form of insurance protects your income in the event of any illness or accident that prevents you from working. The key to permanent health insurance is that the cover (or the payment if you need to claim) is guaranteed until retirement age. This makes it virtually essential insurance for anyone self-employed who does not have similar cover from a company scheme.

As PHI aims at long-term disability the key element is the ability to keep pace with inflation. Should you be unable to work as the result of a car accident or illness which occurs in your early twenties, you need to be confident that your payments 30 years later are still appropriate.

Practice expenses policy

These policies are for people with a dental practice who need to cover basic practice expenses in the event of an accident or illness that prevents them working. Unlike permanent health policies, these policies are usually for a short term (usually 6 or 12 months) because it is likely you will have sold your practice if you are unable to work for longer than 12 months. The fact they are short term means they are much cheaper, especially if they start immediately.

A suggested policy

When considering protecting your income in the event of illness or accident you might well consider a practice expenses policy for 12 months (to cover practice expenses from day one) and a permanent health policy deferred 6 or 12 months (to cover your income in the event of permanent inability to work due to sickness or accident). This is probably the cheapest option, and if you can afford more then deferring the permanent health policy by only 3 months would be sensible as payments would start fairly soon after the cause of the illness or the accident.

However, the sensible move is to obtain appropriate quotes from different companies, making sure you understand the small (but often significant) differences between the different policies. Do not automatically assume that a company or broker with the name 'dentist' in the title is better than all others, no matter what the insurance adviser says. It is always wiser to check for yourself.

Initial banking requirements

Today bank accounts are very different from a decade or so ago, and the choice is so great it can almost be bewildering.

A bank account should be both for convenience and to enable you to earn some interest on your account where possible. Most banks are moving slowly towards internet banking, and although they still have some way to go, we are heading towards a world of digital money without the need for the 'friendly bank manager'.

However, if you are starting a practice you will almost certainly need an overdraft facility, and an understanding bank manager is still worth having. If possible, try to find a bank manager who understands you and there is no harm in 'shopping around' for the best one in your locality.

Once you have set up an account for your business, always keep a separate account for your personal finances. You may decide to have more than one, and often it is wise to keep personal finances in a separate bank, or at least to have different accounts in different banks. If you use telephone or internet banking you can move money from account to account very easily, enabling you to take advantage of different interest rates in the different accounts.

Always be honest in your dealings with the bank. If you know you are going to exceed your overdraft limit then tell the bank, in the hopes they will allow it. If appropriate, visit your bank reasonably frequently when you are setting up and running a practice to keep the bank informed. This is not as necessary as it used to be, but banks like to know that you know what is happening and keep them informed.

Banking is competitive today and it pays to shop around, but be fair in your dealings with your bank as you would expect them to be fair with you.

Further reading

Finance for the Terrified (1998) by Mike Grace. BDJ Books, British Dental Association, 64 Wimpole Street, London W1G 8YS.

All figures are reproduced from the BDJ book Finance for the Terrified by Mike Grace (reproduced with permission).

5.2 MARKETING THE PRACTICE

Practice building is best carried out by word of mouth from satisfied patients recommending the practice to others, rather than by advertising. Similarly, referrals to specialist practices will be made by the general dental practitioner who is satisfied with the treatment provided by a specialist and by the handling of the referred patient.

Minimally invasive techniques, such as those outlined in Section XX are patient friendly, as too are non-intervention preventative techniques. However, the patient needs to be informed that these techniques – as opposed by the outmoded drill and fill philosophy – have been adopted by the practice. This may be by word of mouth at the chairside, by the use of instructional videos, or by patient information leaflets. All staff should be aware of the practice's philosophy, that treatment will not be suggested and carried out unless absolutely essential. A statement to this effect could be included in the practice information leaflet, which should be sent to all new patients in advance of their first appointment. This leaflet should be updated regularly. The setting up of a practice web site may require specialist help, but is possibly the easiest method of communicating the practice philosophy to the public who have access to a computer and modem. The practice web site also requires regular updating. Some practices find that the distribution of a newsletter at regular intervals helps keep the patient base aware of new treatments and practice developments (such as the recruitment of an additional hygienist, for example) and helps put across a caring approach, as well as helping patients identify with *their own* dental practice.

Practice building also means the ability to offer a wide range of treatments. Widening the range of treatments which a dentist can provide usually means attending postgraduate education courses. Patients also need to be made aware of their dentist's commitment to further learning.

Practice marketing is therefore different from traditional marketing of products. The ability to provide a wide range of treatments of high quality at a reasonable cost in a comfortable and caring environment, on a regular basis, is likely to be the best means of 'selling' a practice to its patients.

6 The future

6.1 Career structure in dental practice
6.2 Boredom
6.3 The future

The majority of dental professionals, having spent five years or thereabouts at University, enter practice and remain in that environment for the remainder of their career. While there is always the possibility of a career change within, or outwith, dentistry, there is a potential for stagnation because of the repetitive nature of the job. In this respect, the varied challenges provided by patients are what make life interesting, and a considerable proportion of this book has therefore been dedicated to patient management issues. Striving towards excellence is another way of maintaining interest, and, again, this book has dealt with many issues surrounding this, from planning treatment to minimal intervention. However, it could be considered that the ability to follow a career structure and to take steps to prevent boredom are among the best means to happiness and success in dental practice.

6.1 CAREER STRUCTURE IN DENTAL PRACTICE

While hospital and academic careers have a well-defined career structure, this has not been so, until recently, for general dental practice. The career pathway suggested by the Faculty of General Dental Practitioners (see Chapter 1) provides a suggested career progression, with diplomas being awarded as the candidate progresses. Of course, the incentive to undertake postgraduate diplomas and degrees, which forms part of the promotional pathway for academic and hospital dentists, may not be as strong for general dental practitioners who see no promotion as a result of academic achievement. Nevertheless, practitioners undertake study for further qualifications as a means of enhancing the care of their patients, for mental stimulation and personal achievement.

6.2 BOREDOM

Dental practice has the potential for boredom due to the repetitive nature of some of the work, unless the GDP is aware of this and takes steps to prevent it. These include:

- Developing and maintaining an interest in postgraduate education
- Joining a practice-based research group: these include the Product Research and Evaluation by Practitioners (PREP) Panel, and BRIDGE (Birmingham Research in Dental General Practice) based at the University of Birmingham School of Dentistry, or the Scottish Practice Research Network, based at the Dental school in Dundee. GDPs are uniquely suited to suggest research projects, as the volume of work seen in general dental practice will help the practitioner to identify projects which should be undertaken. Lack of training is not a problem, as dental school staff will invariably be happy to guide the practitioner who is interested.
- Part-time teaching appointments offer the GDP the opportunity to teach his/her potential new colleagues, as well as to mix with the staff in the teaching establishment
- Similarly, part-time clinical assistant positions in hospitals allow the GDP to extend his/her areas of expertise
- Pushing back the frontiers of knowledge by learning new techniques, thereby expanding the areas of clinical expertise. This has two effects, to maintain and improve practice busyness and to force the GDP to work beyond the 'comfort zone'. Developing an interest in dental politics, and representing the profession on committees.

6.3 THE FUTURE

Dental professionals are among the few workers who are unlikely to be replaced by a computer, as patients will remain keen to be treated by a caring human being than by an inanimate computer. However, computers, at the time of writing, are being increasingly employed in a variety of roles in dental practice. These include CAD-CAM manufacture of restorations, the maintenance of patient records and recalls, digital imaging, and the calculation of restoration longevity for clinical governance. Additionally, computers may be utilised to monitor tooth substance loss on digitised casts, and this could be correlated with dietary habits to provide an indication as to whether treatment, or simply monitoring, is needed. All of these could be considered to be more environmentally friendly than 'traditional' practice, as casts, impressions, radiographs and developing solutions are no longer needed. Travel will be reduced by remote diagnosis, with less need to visit referral centres.

Dental disease will continue to be among the most prevalent diseases in the world, albeit reduced when compared with a quarter of a century ago. However, as patients keep their teeth for longer, there will be increasing numbers of teeth in the community which will require inspection, monitoring and treatment. Patients will continue to want their teeth to look good. Dentists will therefore remain busy! The variety of materials which are available to carry out treatment may increase, but not with the near-exponential level of growth seen in the past 25 years. Preventive treatment, which should be funded in the same way as interventive treatment, has always been of relevance, but will take on an increasing role in dental practice, involving an increasing number of PsCD in its implementation.

All of these developments are potentially exciting, ensuring that for the practitioner who maintains his/her interest in their career, dentistry will remain a most rewarding profession.

Index